Management of Primary and Revision Hallux Valgus

Editor

ANDY MOLLOY

FOOT AND ANKLE CLINICS

www.foot.theclinics.com

Consulting Editor
MARK S. MYERSON

June 2014 • Volume 19 • Number 2

ELSEVIER

1600 John F. Kennedy Boulevard ● Suite 1800 ● Philadelphia, Pennsylvania, 19103-2899

http://www.theclinics.com

FOOT AND ANKLE CLINICS Volume 19, Number 2
June 2014 ISSN 1083-7515, ISBN-13: 978-0-323-29920-6

Editor: Jennifer Flynn-Briggs

Foot and Ankle Clinics (ISSN 1083-7515) is published quarterly by Elsevier, Inc., 360 Park Avenue South, New York, NY 10010-1710. Months of issue are March, June, September, and December. Periodicals postage paid at New York, NY, and additional mailing offices. Subscription price per year is $315.00 (US individuals), $421.00 (US institutions), $155.00 (US students), $360.00 (Canadian individuals), $506.00 (Canadian institutions), $215.00 (Canadian students), $460.00 (foreign individuals), $506.00 (foreign institutions), and $215.00 (foreign students). To receive student/resident rate, orders must be accompanied by name of affiliated institution, date of term, and the *signature* of program/residency coordinator on institution letterhead. Orders will be billed at individual rate until proof of status is received. Foreign air speed delivery is included in all *Clinics* subscription prices. All prices are subject to change without notice. **POSTMASTER:** Send address changes to *Foot and Ankle Clinics*, Elsevier Health Sciences Division, Subscription Customer Service, 3251 Riverport Lane, Maryland Heights, MO 63043. **Customer Service: 1-800-654-2452 (US and Canada). From outside of the United States and Canada, call 314-447-8871. Fax: 314-447-8029. E-mail: JournalsCustomerService-usa@ elsevier.com (for print support); JournalsOnlineSupport-usa@elsevier.com (for online support).**

Reprints. For copies of 100 or more, of articles in this publication, please contact the Commercial Reprints Department, Elsevier Inc., 360 Park Avenue South, New York, NY 10010-1710. Tel.: 212-633-3874; Fax: 212-633-3820; E-mail: reprints@elsevier.com.

Contributors

CONSULTING EDITOR

MARK S. MYERSON, MD
Director, The Institute for Foot and Ankle Reconstruction, Mercy Medical Center, Mercy Hospital, Baltimore, Maryland

EDITOR

ANDY MOLLOY, FRCS(Tr&Orth)
Consultant Orthopaedic Surgeon, Orthopaedic Department, University Hospital Aintree, Liverpool, United Kingdom

AUTHORS

CHRIS M. BLUNDELL, MD, FRCS(Orth)
Sheffield Foot and Ankle Unit, Department of Trauma & Orthopaedic Surgery, Sheffield Teaching Hospitals NHS Foundation Trust, Sheffield, United Kingdom

JULIAN CHELL, MBBS, FRCS(Orth)
Consultant Orthopaedic Surgeon, Department of Orthopaedics, Nottingham University Hospitals, City Hospital Campus, Nottingham, United Kingdom

JOSEPH DANIEL, DO
Rothman Institute, Philadelphia, Pennsylvania

MARK B. DAVIES, BM, FRCS(Orth)
Sheffield Foot and Ankle Unit, Department of Trauma & Orthopaedic Surgery, Sheffield Teaching Hospitals NHS Foundation Trust, Sheffield, United Kingdom

SUNIL DHAR, MBBS, MS, MCh Orth, FRCS(Ed Orth)
Consultant Orthopaedic Surgeon, Department of Orthopaedics, Nottingham University Hospitals, City Hospital Campus, Nottingham, United Kingdom

PAULO N. FERRAO, FCS (SA) Ortho
Department of Orthopedic Surgery, WITS University, Johannesburg, South Africa

ANDREW GOLDBERG, MD, FRCS(Tr&Orth)
Consultant Orthopaedic Surgeon, Foot & Ankle Unit, Royal National Orthopaedic Hospital NHS Trust, Stanmore; Clinical Senior Lecturer, UCL Institute of Orthopaedics & Musculoskeletal Science, United Kingdom

MICHAEL S. HENNESSY, BSc, FRCSEd(Tr&Orth)
Consultant Trauma & Orthopaedic Surgeon, Department of Orthopaedics, Wirral University Hospitals NHS Trust, Upton, Wirral, United Kingdom

FABIAN KRAUSE, MD
Department of Orthopaedic Surgery, Inselspital, University of Berne, Bern, Switzerland

ERNESTO MACEIRA, MD
Consultant in Orthopaedic Surgery, Associate Professor of Orthopaedic Surgery, Faculty of Medicine, Universidad Europea Madrid; Orthopaedic Foot and Ankle Unit, Orthopaedic and Trauma Department, Hospital Universitario Quirón Madrid, Madrid, Spain

ADAM G. MILLER, MD
Attending Surgeon, Beacon Orthopaedics and Sports Medicine, Cincinnati, Ohio

ANDY MOLLOY, FRCS(Tr&Orth)
Consultant Orthopaedic Surgeon, Orthopaedic Department, University Hospital Aintree, Liverpool, United Kingdom

MANUEL MONTEAGUDO, MD
Consultant in Orthopaedic Surgery, Associate Professor of Orthopaedic Surgery, Faculty of Medicine, Universidad Europea Madrid; Orthopaedic Foot and Ankle Unit, Orthopaedic and Trauma Department, Hospital Universitario Quirón Madrid, Madrid, Spain

MARK S. MYERSON, MD
Director, The Institute for Foot and Ankle Reconstruction, Mercy Medical Center, Mercy Hospital, Baltimore, Maryland

EZEQUIEL PALMANOVICH, MD
Institute for the Foot and Ankle Reconstruction, Mercy Hospital, Baltimore, Maryland

ANTHONY MICHAEL PERERA, FRCS(Orth)
London Foot & Ankle Centre, Hospital St John & St Elizabeth, London; Spire Cardiff Hospital, Cardiff, United Kingdom

STEVEN M. RAIKIN, MD
Professor Orthopaedic Surgery, Director, Foot and Ankle Service, Rothman Institute, Philadelphia, Pennsylvania

DAVID REDFERN, FRCS(Tr&Orth)
London Foot & Ankle Centre, Hospital St John & St Elizabeth, London, United Kingdom

NIKIFOROS P. SARAGAS, FCS (SA) Ortho, MMed (Ortho Surg)(Wits)
Department of Orthopedic Surgery, WITS University, Johannesburg, South Africa

TIMO SCHMID, MD
Department of Orthopaedic Surgery, Inselspital, University of Berne, Bern, Switzerland

DISHAN SINGH, FRCS(Orth)
Consultant Orthopaedic Surgeon, Foot & Ankle Unit, Royal National Orthopaedic Hospital NHS Trust, Stanmore, United Kingdom

CHRISTOPHER R. WALKER, MCH(Orth), FRCS(Orth), FRCS(Eng), FRCS(Ed)
Consultant in Trauma & Orthopaedic Surgery, Department of Orthopaedics, Royal Liverpool University Hospital, Liverpool, United Kingdom

JAMES WIDNALL, MRCS
Orthopaedic Registrar, Orthopaedic Department, University Hospital Aintree, Liverpool, United Kingdom

EDWARD V. WOOD, FRCS(Tr&Orth)
Consultant Trauma & Orthopaedic Surgeon, Department of Orthopaedics, Countess of Chester Hospital NHS Trust, Chester, United Kingdom

Contents

Rotational osteotomies such as the Ludloff and proximal opening wedge have not been popular historically because of instability from lack of fixation, resulting in complications. This article describes modified techniques with modern fixation of these 2 osteotomies, which offer stable fixation and reproducible results.

Due to its proximal correction site and long lever arm, the Lapidus fusion, modified or not, is a powerful technique to correct hallux valgus deformities. The disadvantages are a high complication rate and a long postoperative rehabilitation period. It is only performed in 5% to 10% of all hallux valgus deformity corrections but remains, however, an important procedure, especially in moderate to severe deformities with intermetatarsal angles more than 14°, hypermobility of the first ray, arthritis of the first tarsometatarsal joint, and recurrent deformities. This article provides an overview of the procedure with special focus on the surgical technique.

Hallux valgus in children is a relatively uncommon deformity, also known by several other names such as juvenile or adolescent bunion, metatarsus primus varus, and metatarsus primus adductus. The presence of an open growth plate is considered by most to be part of the definition of this condition. However, others include patients up to age 20 years, owing to the plastic nature of the various components of the condition. The presenting complaint is invariably of the bunion and its cosmetic appearance. Treatment should be conservative and surgery avoided till skeletal maturity is achieved due to the high incidence of recurrence in children.

Arthrodesis of the first metatarsophalangeal joint is a reliable operation in the treatment of selected cases of hallux valgus. It corrects deformity of hallux valgus and metatarsus primus varus, leading to good functional results with a low complication rate. It is a technique well suited to patients with hallux valgus associated with degenerative changes or severe deformity, and those for whom primary hallux valgus surgery has failed.

Recurrence of hallux valgus deformity can be a common complication after corrective surgery. The cause of recurrent hallux valgus is usually multifactorial, and includes patient-related factors such as preoperative anatomic predisposition, medical comorbidities, compliance with postcorrection instructions, and surgical factors such as choice of the appropriate procedure and technical competency. For a successful outcome, this cause must be ascertained preoperatively. Although the algorithm to determine which intervention should be used is not unlike that of primary hallux valgus surgery, operative correction of hallux valgus recurrence can be challenging. This article discusses these challenges, complications, causes, and techniques.

FOOT AND ANKLE CLINICS

ISSUE OF RELATED INTEREST

Medical Clinics of North America March 2014 (Vol. 98, Issue 2)
Managing and Treating Common Foot and Ankle Problems
John A. DiPreta, *Editor*
Available at: http://www.medical.theclinics.com/

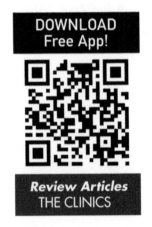

NOW AVAILABLE FOR YOUR iPhone and iPad

Preface

Management of Primary and Revision Hallux Valgus

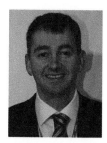

Andy Molloy, FRCS(Tr&Orth)
Editor

Hallux valgus is one of the most common conditions we treat as foot and ankle orthopedic surgeons. It can have significant impact on patients' lives through effects on stance, walking, sporting activity, and ability to fit into footwear. It represents a large spectrum of pathologic abnormality ranging from the pediatric hallux valgus to the development of secondary arthritic changes. As with all surgery, there are a range of complications, including recurrence, varus, and shortening.

The authors of this edition of *Foot and Ankle Clinics of North America* are experts in dealing with hallux valgus. The articles deal with primary pathologic abnormality, from mild to severe deformities in both adults and children, as well as the role of fusion surgery. This issue also deals with the extremely challenging topic of revision surgery, delineating the underlying pathologic abnormalities and surgical strategies for correcting them. I would like to commend and thank the authors for their outstanding contributions for making this an excellent and complete overview of hallux valgus surgery. I would also like to thank the staff at Elsevier for their help in putting together this issue.

Mark Myerson has been a true friend and a fantastic mentor over the years for which I am extremely thankful and grateful. He deserves our recognition and thanks in constantly pushing the boundaries and developing orthopedic foot and ankle surgery as well as his tireless efforts in education and research.

I sincerely hope you enjoy this issue of *Foot and Ankle Clinics of North America* and that it is of great help in treating your patients for what is frequently a challenging condition.

Andy Molloy, FRCS(Tr&Orth)
University Hospital Aintree
Lower Lane
Liverpool, L9 7AL, UK

E-mail address:
andymolloy3@gmail.com

Foot Ankle Clin N Am 19 (2014) ix
http://dx.doi.org/10.1016/j.fcl.2014.03.002
1083-7515/14/$ – see front matter © 2014 Elsevier Inc. All rights reserved.

foot.theclinics.com

Scarf Osteotomy

Andy Molloy, FRCS(Tr&Orth)*, James Widnall, MRCS

KEYWORDS

• Hallux valgus • Bunion • Scarf • Osteotomy • Metatarsal

KEY POINTS

- The scarf osteotomy is an extremely powerful and versatile method of correcting hallux valgus.
- Scarf osteotomy can be used to correct a large range of deformities, including an altered distal metatarsal articular angle.
- As with all operations, complications may arise, but the rate can be diminished by accurate preoperative planning and osteotomy technique.

ETIOLOGY

Both extrinsic and intrinsic factors have been reported as causative factors in hallux valgus. Various studies have shown that shoe wearing significantly increases the prevalence of the deformity.[1–3] Work by Sim-Fook and Hodgson[3] in the 1950s showed a 33% association between shoe wearing and hallux valgus (compared with 2% in the bare-footed population). High heels have also been attributed to the deformity[4] with the rationale of increased first-ray loading as the foot slides forward into the toe box being suggested as the main driving force.[5] It is deemed, however, that this increased forefoot loading is likely to be more influential in progression rather than initiation of deformity.[6] Other causes of increased forefoot loading, such as occupation, obesity, and excessive walking, have not been shown to have a causative link with hallux valgus.[7–10]

Intrinsic factors also feature, with genetics being a forerunner. Articles have quoted between 68% and 90% of affected patients showing a familial tendency.[11,12] It has been documented that gender is also a significant factor. It is well known that women are far more likely to seek surgical treatment for their hallux valgus deformity (female to male ratio 15:1).[13,14] However, it is unclear as to how much this ratio is influenced by the increased prevalence of abnormality (owing to a higher prevalence of laxity and first-ray hypermobility)[15,16] being secondary to gender, and the increased tendency for women to wear high-heeled or poorly fitting shoes.[17,18]

A large body of work has been published regarding pes planus and its role in hallux valgus. It is thought that although it probably does not initiate the deformity it seems to

Orthopaedic Department, University Hospital Aintree, Lower Lane, Liverpool L9 7AL, UK
* Corresponding author.
E-mail address: andymolloy3@gmail.com

Foot Ankle Clin N Am 19 (2014) 165–180
http://dx.doi.org/10.1016/j.fcl.2014.02.001
1083-7515/14/$ – see front matter © 2014 Elsevier Inc. All rights reserved.

increase the rate of progression,[19] which is explained primarily by the increased loading on the medial border of the hallux secondary to excessive pronation.[20] However, it should be noted that pes planus has not been shown to have a negative effect on outcomes following surgery for hallux valgus.[16,21]

First-ray hypermobility has been reported to be responsible for hallux valgus.[22,23] A positive correlation has been shown between hallux valgus and first-ray hypermobility.[24] There are also several studies that have shown stabilization of the tarsometatarsal joint (TMTJ), without fusion, following first-ray realignment procedures.[25,26] This finding leads to the conclusion that hypermobility may be secondary to a decrease in soft-tissue stability as opposed to being a primary force behind the hallux valgus deformity.[27] The other confounding factor in this debate is the lack of clinical correlation in determining how one accurately delineates first-ray hypermobility.[24]

The windlass mechanism is another deforming force in hallux valgus. On weight bearing, the hallux valgus deformity is increased owing to the tightening of the plantar fascia and concurrent pronation.[28] On activation of the windlass mechanism on heel raise, the first metatarsophalangeal joint (MTPJ) has to reciprocally dorsiflex. Tightening the plantar fascia exerts an opposing force to the ground reaction force on the MTPJ. These opposing forces result in the hallux following the path of least resistance and a subsequent increase in deformity.[29] It has been proposed that first-ray hypermobility may be partially explained by transmission of these forces through a rigid MTPJ.[30]

PATHOANATOMY

It is thought that hallux valgus deformity follows a stepwise deterioration.[31,32] Critically the medial structures (medial sesamoid and medial collateral ligaments) of the MTPJ must fail.[33] This failure permits varus movement of the metatarsal, which can be exacerbated by instability at TMTJ. The proximal phalanx responds by a relative valgus movement attributable to its attachments to the phalangeosesamoid ligament, the plantar plate, and adductor hallucis. The resulting position of the metatarsal head leads to erosion of the cartilage covering the medial sesamoid as well as the nearby crista. When coupled with weakness of the medial sesamoid ligament, the deformity can progress rapidly.[29] The lateral sesamoid tends to be left uncovered as the head of the metatarsal slips from its original position overlying the sesamoid apparatus.[19] Owing to the medial prominence, the overlying bursa thickens as it is subjected to abnormally high pressures from footwear. The deformity then progresses as the long flexors and extensors acting on the hallux function as adductors as they bowstring laterally.[34] Secondary to the pull of adductor hallucis and lateral head of flexor hallucis brevis, combined with the dysfunction of the medial musculature (medial head of flexor hallucis brevis and abductor hallucis), the first metatarsal pronates, resulting in offloading of the first ray onto the lesser toes.[35] This process can result in lesser toe clawing and associated metatarsophalangeal subluxation.

TECHNIQUE

The first descriptions of a z-shaped osteotomy were by Burutaran[36] and Zygmunt.[37] However, the term scarf osteotomy was first used by Weil, who presented results from more than 1000 cases.[38] Scarf is a carpentry term describing beveling the ends of 2 pieces of wood and securely fastening them so that they overlap to create one continuous piece. This technique was popularized by Weil[38,39] and Barouk[40,41] as a versatile method of correcting hallux valgus while maintaining the blood supply to the metatarsal head. It also has rigid fixation, allowing early mobilization.

The indications for the use of a scarf osteotomy are hallux valgus of up to and including severe deformities. However, one must ensure that there is sufficient width of metatarsal to allow correction (see later discussion). Contraindications include the presence of ongoing infection, moderate to severe arthritis of the first MTPJ or first TMTJ, and frank hypermobility of the first TMTJ.

Patients are seen 2 to 3 weeks preoperatively by a specialist nurse and physiotherapist. All aspects of the operation and postoperative care are reiterated to the patient, having already been previously covered during the consent process when listed for surgery in the outpatient clinic. The patients are then assessed for their ability to bear weight as tolerated. Appropriate practice instruction and advice are given so that the patients have thoroughly practiced their level of mobilization, enabling a smooth same-day discharge. This routine has led to a significant reduction in stay.[42]

In the authors' institution most patients are operated on under general anesthetic, although regional anesthesia may be used. A single dose of intravenous antibiotics is given on induction. A local anesthetic ankle block is performed using 10 mL each of short-lasting and long-lasting local anesthetic. The patient is positioned supine and a thigh tourniquet is used.

Before commencing the operation, the authors consider it essential that the osteotomy is templated, meaning that an accurate preoperative plan is made to ensure that the correct deformity correction is performed. The length of the osteotomy, the direction of the transverse limbs, and the required amount of translation are determined. The length of the osteotomy will be determined by the amount of translation required. The authors would recommend that the maximum translation that can be aimed for is approximately 75% of the diameter of the shaft, which will allow at least cortex to cortex contact along the length of the osteotomy. The osteotomy is then made as long as necessary to allow this amount of translation, while ensuring that the proximal part of the osteotomy does not exit in the vessels on the plantar aspect of the neck. Therefore, most of the time a shorter scarf can be performed (3–3.5 cm), which only goes into the metaphysis. However, if a larger degree of translation is required then it may need to extend proximally into the start of the diaphyseal flare, as this will give a larger surface area for translation.

The authors perform the operation standing on the same side that is being operated on, turning the leg into external rotation. This positioning is helpful in ensuring that the correct plantarflexed direction of the longitudinal limb is achieved.

The lateral release is a crucial step of the operation. For the most severe deformities, this release is performed in what can be considered the standard fashion. A dorsal longitudinal incision of approximately 2.5 cm is performed in the first interspace, centered around the level of the first MTPJ. Blunt dissection is then performed down to the side of the first metatarsal. A self-retaining retractor is then inserted as deep as possible, tensioning the tissues in the first interspace. A scalpel is then inserted vertically against the lateral part of the neck of the first metatarsal as deep as the cutting edge of a #12 blade with the cutting edge facing distally. The blade is then swept distally, staying against bone, up to approximately 5 mm onto the shaft on the proximal phalanx. The blade is the rotated 45° laterally, and a small (approximately 5 mm) sweep is performed to ensure that the lateral structures are released without damaging the neurovascular bundle. If the fibular sesamoid is particularly retracted and rotated, the proximal and lateral sides of the sesamoid are circumcised to enable reduction. For lesser deformities the lateral release is carried out in a different fashion (see later discussion).

The medial skin incision is performed with the proximal phalanx being held parallel to the shaft of the first metatarsal, enabling a straight incision to be performed. The length of the incision is determined by the preoperative plan. Blunt dissection is then performed to ensure that the medial cutaneous nerve is not within the operative field. Once safe, the scalpel is placed directly against bone on the proximal phalanx and a longitudinal capsulotomy is performed extending as far proximally as has been determined by the preoperative plan. Subperiosteal dissection is then performed, using long strokes, ensuring that a good-quality cuff of capsular tissue is present for capsulorrhaphy. It is imperative that this dissection completely avoids the plantar aspect of the metatarsal neck, as this is the only completely intact significant blood supply to the metatarsal head (**Fig. 1**). This dissection, however, is extended over to the lateral side of the shaft of the metatarsal, as removal of this periosteum will make translation of the osteotomy easier. If not previously performed, the lateral release can now be made over the top of the metatarsal. A little of the dorsal capsule at the base of the proximal phalanx will need to be elevated. An elevator is inserted vertically past the lateral side of the head, which will allow good visualization of the deforming lateral structures and allow the lateral release to be performed under direct vision by the same method as previously described. The authors find that this technique is highly effective in most moderate to severe deformities, and provides better cosmesis by avoiding the dorsal first web incision. In the most severe deformities adequate visualization can be difficult. It is of paramount importance that the release is adequate, and if not sure the surgeon should then revert to the standard technique.

The scarf osteotomy is powerful, and therefore needs to be carried out with as much precision as possible. For this reason the authors remove a sliver off the medial eminence, which provides a flat surface against which to perform the scarf osteotomy, helping prevent chattering of the saw blade. However, it is essential that this resection is minimal. Resection reduces the width of the metatarsal head and, therefore, the available diameter for translation and obtaining fixation. The resection is done with a saw going from just medial to the sulcus, and is taken proximally, so that the cut is virtually planar with the medial side of the first metatarsal shaft.

The scarf osteotomy is then marked using electrocautery. The distal apex is at the junction of the dorsal one-third and plantar two-thirds of the head just proximal to the cartilage of the joint (normally approximately 7 mm from the joint surface). The proximal apex of the osteotomy will be at the junction of the dorsal two-thirds and plantar one-third of the shaft. For those who are inexperienced, it is helpful to score this line with the saw. The coronal alignment of the longitudinal limb should be plantar, so that the head of the metatarsal is plantarflexed on translation. A plantarflexed cut also helps resists troughing caused by the direction of forces put through the cancellous

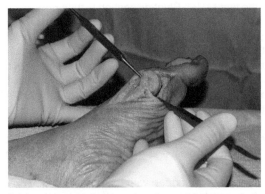

Fig. 1. Dissection of the metatarsal, leaving the plantar blood supply intact.

bone. The correct angle can be determined by resting the saw blade against the proximal plantar aspect of the shaft. Elevators are used as retractors; one vertically against the lateral part of the neck with the second horizontally on the plantar aspect of the metatarsal head. The osteotomy is then performed, going from distal to proximal. The authors find it easier, thereby reducing troughing, to insert the saw up to the lateral cortex along the length of the osteotomy, and then to use this initial cut as a guide for breaching the lateral cortex.

The distal transverse limb is then performed. As previously mentioned, to keep the first metatarsal at the same relative length the osteotomy is performed perpendicular to the second metatarsal shaft. The osteotomy can be used to shorten the first metatarsal by heading more proximal to this line and vice versa. The easiest way to mark this limb is by marking it out on the preoperative template and continuing the line over to the lateral border of the foot so that there is an anatomic landmark to head for. The transverse limb should run just proximal to the cartilage of the metatarsal head. The other line of orientation is the angle of the transverse limb compared with the longitudinal one, looking at the medial side of the shaft. This angle should be 70° to 80°. The authors do not think that this gives the osteotomy inherent stability (or it would not need to be fixed), but it does help in providing control when applying translational force. An elevator is placed as a retractor in the previous position so as to protect the neurovascular bundle. The most frequent cause of not fully connecting these 2 limbs of the osteotomy is that the saw is not angled enough in a plantar direction.

The proximal transverse limb should then be performed. It is imperative that this is performed parallel to the distal transverse limb. If not, translation will not be possible. In this eventuality, a 1-mm sliver of bone should be taken of the proximal plantar part of the metatarsal to provide enough room for translation to be performed. When connecting the limbs of the osteotomy, great care should be taken not to crosshatch, as this may precipitate a fracture. When first starting to use the scarf osteotomy, crosshatching can be prevented by inserting a 1-mm wire into the medial side of the shaft of the first metatarsal at each of the apices.

The osteotomy should open up with no force applied if the osteotomy has been fully completed. It should not be levered apart because this has a high chance of causing a fracture, especially distally in the head. If is not fully opening and its completeness has been checked with the saw, there is usually some lateral periosteum holding the 2 fragments together. An elevator should be inserted through the osteotomy to free this up (without levering) (**Fig. 2**).

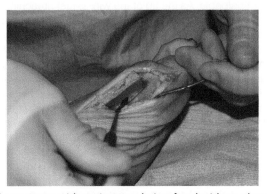

Fig. 2. Completed osteotomy with periosteum being freed with an elevator.

The aim of the osteotomy is translate the head laterally into the correct anatomic position. Care should therefore be taken that this happens, rather than pulling on the shaft so that this moves medially and the head remains in the same position. This action is taken by holding the medial distal corner of the dorsal shaft with a pointed clip in a static position and pushing the head laterally with the thumb. The amount of translation should be the same distance as measured in the preoperative plan. If there is a grossly altered distal metatarsal articular angle (DMAA), this can be corrected by adding rotation to translation of the osteotomy. A medial-based 1-mm wedge is usually sufficient and is taken from both ends of the dorsal part of the osteotomy. The same maneuver as previously described is undertaken, as well as using an elevator to press against the most proximal plantar part of the osteotomy to achieve the desired rotation as determined by directed visualization of the metatarsal head.

The translated osteotomy is the provisionally held with two 1-mm wires. The distal one is the first to be inserted. It is placed approximately 7 mm from the distal transverse limb so that the head of the screw will not fracture out through it. It should be placed at the same oblique angle as the distal transverse limb in the sagittal plane. It should also be a close as possible to the new anatomic axis of the first metatarsal in the axial plane. If it is oblique to this, translation will be lost as compression from the screw is applied. Care should also be taken that it is not so close as to breech the lateral cortex. The wire should then be inserted so that the tip of the wire just breeches the articular surface of the metatarsal head. The proximal wire is then inserted approximately 7 mm from the proximal end of the osteotomy. If there has been rotation of the osteotomy, it will need to be placed more distally. The wire is placed as vertically as possible toward the lateral side of the shaft. If the screw is placed obliquely, it will obviously be very oblique to the plantar part of the osteotomy and will not obtain sufficient purchase. If an elevator is placed under the plantar surface, one should be able to visually confirm that the wire has engaged both sides of the osteotomy and is sitting approximately 2 mm outside the cortex. The appearance should then be checked clinically and fluoroscopically. The authors have previously demonstrated that using fluoroscopy adds significant accuracy to the position achieved.[43] One should check that the metatarsal head is seated over the sesamoids, the intermetatarsal and hallux valgus angles are corrected, and there has been no inadvertent lengthening or shortening of the first metatarsal. One should also be able to achieve as close to possible to 60° to 90° of dorsiflexion.

If the appearance is satisfactory, the wires are measured for screw length. The distal screw is a unicortical screw. The authors use headless compression screws so that the screw head is not palpable. As the tip of the wire is just breeching the articular surface, 6 mm is subtracted from the measured length to ensure that the screw tip is not in the joint. The screw hole is then drilled, ensuring that the surgeon has the thumb firmly inserted against the medial side of the head, because the drilled screw hole can allow some rotation of the osteotomy and cause some loss of position. The drill should be fully inserted so that the screw head is fully drilled. If not, a fracture may be precipitated. The screw is then inserted. The proximal screw should be inserted at the same length as the wire measures. However, if it is difficult to directly visualize the tip of proximal wire, 2 mm should be taken off the length of the wire, as it is easy to insert the wire a little long. Normally the proximal screw is 2 to 4 mm shorter than the distal one. The proximal wire is then overdrilled. The assistant should have a hemostat to hand, as this wire usually comes out with the drill. Again it is imperative that the surgeon has the thumb against the osteotomy so that position is not lost. The screw is then inserted. The medial overhang of the osteotomy is then excised with a saw.

It is helpful to ensure that there are no sharp angular edges because although they will remodel with time, they can be initially a little uncomfortable for patients.

It is the authors' firm belief that if there is any hallux interphalangeus or any residual valgus present (providing that the head is in a good position and the lateral release is complete), an Akin osteotomy should be performed. A capsulorrhaphy alone should not be relied on, as it is easy to tip the hallux into varus or, more commonly, for recurrent valgus to ensue.

The Akin osteotomy is performed at the junction of the diaphysis and the metaphyseal flare at the base of the proximal phalanx. The skin incision should be lengthened to just distal to this level. Ensuring no damage to medial nerves, a scalpel is inserted over the dorsal and plantar surfaces of the phalanx with the blade parallel to these surfaces. Just enough room should be created to allow curved edges of elevators to be inserted as retractors to protect the extensor and flexor tendons. Standard oscillating saw blades remove approximately 1 mm of bone. Therefore, the maximum wedge that should be excised is approximately 1 mm. In small deformities no wedge of bone will be necessary. The osteotomy should be performed leaving the lateral cortex intact so that control of the osteotomy can be maintained. If a wedge is excised, one should ensure that excision is complete. It is most common to leave small fragments in the plantar aspect of the osteotomy, which can be removed with a hemostat. The osteotomy is then closed manually. The osteotomy is usually fixed with a headless compression screw, as the authors find this to be the most reliable and reproducible method. A 1-mm wire is therefore inserted from the medial corner of the proximal phalanx, just distal to the articular surface at approximately 45° to the mechanical axis. The clinically and fluoroscopically correct position is confirmed, and the screw of appropriate size inserted.

The authors use imbrication of the capsule as the method of capsulorrhaphy. If there has been a particularly large correction, the redundant skin and capsule are excised. However, one needs to ensure that sufficient good-quality capsule is left so that the stitches do not pull out. Three horizontal mattress sutures are used with a heavy absorbable suture. The sutures are placed from in to out so that the knots are buried. A couple of subcutaneous sutures are used to oppose the skin, and a running nonabsorbable suture is used for the skin. A nonadhesive dressing that has longitudinal cut in it is applied, so that 2 small pieces of Velband can be inserted to help splint the hallux. A bandage is then applied.

The patients are usually discharged on the same day, weight bearing as tolerated, in a standard postoperative shoe, with an advice leaflet on mobilization and exercises. Patients are seen at 2 weeks for removal of sutures. No splintage is applied to the hallux, and patients have active and passive exercises reiterated to them. Patients are then assessed clinically and radiologically at 6 weeks (**Fig. 3**), after which they are allowed to don their own appropriate footwear.

RESULTS

Surgical correction of hallux valgus has been demonstrated to be an effective treatment modality in comparison with conservative treatment.[44] Since Barouk's original article,[40] the main advantages of a scarf osteotomy over other surgical techniques have been stated as being its versatility, early functional recovery, preservation of the first MTPJ motion, and long-term reliability. Much work has been done, albeit in mostly small numbers, in an attempt to scrutinize Barouk's technique in the clinical setting. Outcomes have traditionally been clinical and radiographic measures. More recently, pedobarography has also been used. Clinical measures tend to include

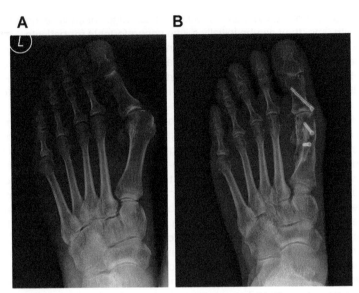

Fig. 3. (*A*) Preoperative and (*B*) postoperative radiographs of hallux valgus corrected with scarf osteotomy.

clinical appearance, foot posture, range of motion at the MTPJ, and recurrence of the deformity. Such variables are mostly covered by the American Orthopaedic Foot and Ankle Society (AOFAS) Hallux Metatarsophalangeal Interphalangeal Scale,[45] which is the most commonly used scoring system. Radiographically the use of weight-bearing anteroposterior and lateral radiographs permit the measurement of the hallux valgus angle (HVA), intermetatarsal angle (IMA), DMAA, and the medial sesamoid position. Pedobarographic studies can then be used to measure changes in peak pressure, mean pressure, pressure/time, and force/time.[46]

Lipscombe and colleagues[46] agreed with Barouk's early conclusions, at least in the mid term. Thirty-one feet underwent scarf osteotomies for the treatment of hallux valgus. In the prospective follow-up radiographic, clinical, and pedobarographic assessments were performed. Union was achieved both radiographically and clinically at 6 weeks in all patients. AOFAS scores showed a significant (*P*<.01) average increase from 47.94 to 96.10 at 12 months postoperatively. This subjective decrease in symptoms was shown to have been maintained at 5 years after surgery according to a modified (nonvalidated) AOFAS questionnaire. Both the HVA and IMA were improved significantly. No notable difference was shown by pedobarographic studies.

An earlier, retrospective study by Crevoisier and colleagues[47] echoed the increase in patient satisfaction, again with the use of AOFAS scores (*P*<.001). Weight-bearing radiographs showed significant changes in HVA and IMA. The Hardy-Clapham score[48] (medial sesamoid position) also improved (*P*<.001). Interestingly the investigators contradicted Barouk's original point on preserved MTPJ motion, with 7% of patients exhibiting a decreased range of movement at the average 22-month follow-up. An Akin procedure was performed in 71% (60 of 84) of operations. No difference in outcome, clinical or radiographic, was demonstrated in patients with multiple procedures.

The early return to function for patients having undergone a scarf osteotomy was highlighted by Kristen and colleagues[49] study, with an average return to work at

5.8 weeks and a return to sport at 8.3 weeks. The previously documented increase in AOFAS forefoot scores and HVA/IMA changes were also seen (P<.001).

Adding further ballast to Barouk's early comments, Lorei and colleagues[50] reported results adding to the positive body of work behind the scarf technique. Postoperative AOFAS scores were at an average of 89. No preoperative scores were recorded for comparison. Contrary to Crevoisier and colleagues,[47] these investigators demonstrated an increase in first MTPJ range of movement from 59.7° to 71.1° (P<.001). Radiographic analysis showed significant changes in HVA (32.5° to 6.2°), IMA (15.5° to 6.6°), and medial sesamoid position (P<.001). Moreover, pedobarographic testing showed relatively normal postoperative foot loading, with a postoperative increase in medial forefoot loading at the average 33-month follow-up.

Jones and colleagues[51] also performed a prospective pedobarographic outcome study. Thirty-five feet underwent a scarf osteotomy of the first metatarsal and Akin osteotomy procedure. Using method of pedobarographic data collection of Betts and colleagues,[52] they recorded a change of the first metatarsal head peak pressure between preoperative and postoperative measurements, although this was not significant (P = .2). The mean readings both preoperatively and postoperatively were within the normal range. No difference was seen between the preoperatively and postoperative measurements on the nonoperated feet in patients who underwent unilateral procedures. Two patients were shown to have increased first metatarsal head pressures; one had a low AOFAS score and was not content with the surgical outcome. The other had a long distal screw subsequently removed. A mean improvement of 6° and 19° was seen in the IMA and HVA, respectively. No significant change was noted in the DMAA. The first MTPJ range of motion increased in 26% of cases and remained static in a further 63%.

Similar improvements in the clinical status, AOFAS score, and radiographic evaluation have been shown in several publications, indicating predictable and positive results for scarf-corrected hallux valgus deformities.[53–57]

The application of the scarf is not limited to adults. George and colleagues[58] retrospectively examined its use in adolescent hallux valgus correction whereby 19 feet underwent a scarf osteotomy. At 6 weeks after surgery there was a significant improvement in the IMA, HVA, and DMAA (P<.0001). Unfortunately, by the average follow-up of 37.6 months the change in both the DMAA and HVA, when compared with preoperative radiographs, was no longer significant (P = .32). The changes in IMA remained significant until the study's conclusion. Because of this recurrence, the investigators recommended deferring the use of a scarf osteotomy as treatment of hallux valgus until skeletal maturity has been reached.

The scarf technique has been compared with other surgical options. In a recent meta-analysis[59] of 1351 feet, the scarf (n = 300) was compared with the chevron osteotomy (n = 1028). The sole outcome measurement was the postoperative reduction of the IMA. The chevron cohort demonstrated an average decrease of 5.33°. The scarf group held a significant 0.88° larger reduction (P<.001), with an average decrease in the IMA of 6.21°. However, this apparent 1° extra correction offered by the scarf may be explained by the difference in the preoperative IMA between the 2 groups (13.2° chevron; 14.3° scarf). This difference may well have led to bias with regard to the selected operative technique. It should also be noted that the investigators deduced that many of the studies included in the meta-analysis were of a low quality according to the GRADE system.

Dhukaram and colleagues[60] compared the Mitchell osteotomy with scarf osteotomy in 28 patients. Each cohort consisted of 22 feet. A control group of 20 feet was also used for comparison in pedobarographic testing. The postoperative AOFAS scores at an average of 27 months of follow-up showed the scarf cohort to exhibit higher clinical scores when compared with the Mitchell osteotomy group (84 vs 74). The investigators analyzed mean pressure, peak pressure, and total contact time using pedobarographic testing. Both groups exhibited reduced pressure distribution under the hallux when compared with the controls, with the scarf group being less affected. However, the pressure distribution under the first metatarsal head was comparable with that of the controls. The Mitchell cohort had increased loading over the second and third metatarsal heads, with the scarf group overloading the heel and midfoot. There was a significant correlation between hallux pressure readings and positive AOFAS scores. The investigators concluded that there was a better outcome with increasing loads through the hallux.

More recently, the scarf has also been compared favorably with an arthrodesis of the first MTPJ. Desmarchelier and colleagues[61] compared the functional results of isolated procedures in 50 patients. Clinical evaluation was carried out using the AOFAS, 36-Item Short-Form (SF-36), Foot Function Index (FFI), and the Foot and Ankle Ability Measure (FAAM). Both cohorts were comparable with respect to overall satisfaction (90% arthrodesis; 91.4% scarf) and pain (AOFAS pain score 35.6 vs 34.5). However, significant functional differences were demonstrated in all scoring systems in favor of the scarf (SF-36 62.3 vs 70.9; FFI 19.8 vs 8.6; FAAM 87% vs 94%). One major potential for bias is the difference of indication for surgery in each cohort, as well as the fact that there is no movement at the first MTPJ after an arthrodesis. There was, however, no difference between hallux valgus and hallux rigidus in the arthrodesis group.

Unfortunately, most current work lacks impact because of the relatively low patient numbers. For future work to permit meta-analysis and to allow complete evaluation of the scarf procedure, follow-up needs to be multifaceted, including clinical, radiologic, and pedobarographic data. Despite this, the scarf technique has been shown to produce effective and reproducible relief from symptomatic hallux valgus in even the most severe deformities (**Fig. 4**).

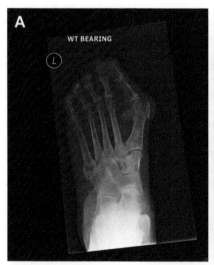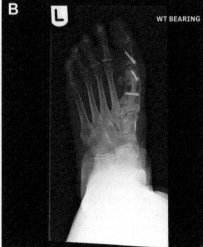

Fig. 4. (*A*) Preoperative and (*B*) postoperative radiographs of correction of a severe hallux valgus.

COMPLICATIONS

Despite having good published results,[46,62,63] the surgical correction of hallux valgus with a scarf osteotomy is not without limitations. It has been documented to possess a steep learning curve,[41] and complications have been reported to range anywhere between 6% and 35%.[64,65]

The potential complications may be intraoperative or postoperative. Intraoperative issues were highlighted by Smith and colleagues,[64] who identified first metatarsal fracture (3%) and Kirschner-wire shearing (1%) as their most commonly encountered problems. The risk of metatarsal fracturing was noted, albeit anecdotally, to be associated with attempted displacement with incomplete osteotomies and inadequate countersinking from the graduated Barouk drill bit. Ensuring that the wider-diameter portion of the drill is fully flush with the cortex should prevent excess stress at the point of screw insertion.

Elsewhere, intraoperative troughing has been shown to be a prevalent complication. Coetzee[65] reported troughing, with loss of metatarsal height, in 35% of cases. Troughing results in offloading of the first ray owing to excessive pronation and subsequent overload of lesser toes. It was suggested that careful patient selection of younger individuals with healthier bone and a 3-mm limit of the distal and proximal step cut could minimize the risk of troughing. A rotational malunion can often be seen secondary to the effect of troughing, and has been reported by the same author to be as high as 30% of all cases. The resulting deformity was reported to be very difficult to rectify.

Shortening of the metatarsal is caused by the transverse limbs of the osteotomy being carried out at an angle of less than 90° to the second metatarsal shaft. In some circumstances, it can be of benefit to the surgeon, and highlights the versatility of technique. Inadvertent shortening will make the lesser metatarsal relatively too long and will therefore increase load through them, promoting callosity formation and transfer metatarsalgia. However, inadvertent shortening is thought to be less of a problem with the scarf than with other first metatarsal osteotomies.[64]

The postoperative period is also open to complications. Stress fractures have been highlighted since Barouk's original article[41] and have been noted in numerous subsequent studies.[64,65] It is thought that they are usually secondary to suboptimal distal screw placement. Alterations to Barouk's original technique, such as decreasing the obliquity of the distal transverse cut to 80°, as opposed to 60°,[64] have also been suggested to decrease the risk of later stress fractures, in conjunction with meticulous screw placement. The result of stress fracture of the distal first metatarsal can result in elevation of the first ray, leading to transfer metatarsalgia. It has been recommended to treat such cases with heel-support shoes, removal of the distal screw, and Weil metatarsal osteotomies if transfer metatarsalgia persists.[41]

Avascular necrosis of the metatarsal head has been shown to be a late complication. Owing to the nature of the soft-tissue dissection the operating surgeon must be aware, and actively preserve, the predominant plantar blood supply to the metatarsal head. Lipscombe and colleagues[46] reported 1 case from the 31 in their study. Treatment consisted of removal of metalwork and subsequent arthrodesis of the MTPJ. However, this complication can only arise from inadvertent dissection under the plantar aspect of the neck or if the patient has a plantar blood supply that is relatively insignificant. Fortunately, this is an extremely rare complication. The other significant complication in this series was that of a traumatic neuroma (2 of 31 cases; 6.45%), which was managed conservatively with orthotics.

Neuralgic symptoms also featured in the study by Crevoisier and colleagues.[47] Three cases (out of 84 feet) suffered postoperative neuralgia in the first web space, which was deduced to be due to their open lateral release. The investigators therefore advocated performing lateral release through the medial incision. All 3 cases had recovered spontaneously by 6 months postoperatively. Four patients (4.8%) suffered from persisting scar tenderness.

Persistent pain can also be caused by prominent metalwork, most notably the distal screw. Jones and colleagues[51] reported 1 case (2.9%) of persistent pain on weight bearing. Radiographs revealed a proud screw, which was subsequently removed to settle the patient's symptoms. Other investigators have had similar experiences (**Fig. 5**).[46,47]

Because of the shape of the scarf osteotomy, the stability of intraoperative fixation, and the large area of the osteotomy, an environment suited to primary bone healing is created, which permits early weight bearing in an attempt to prevent long-standing MTPJ stiffness.[37] However, cases of unstable fixation have been published. Two of 84 feet were found to have unstable fixation in one study.[47] One case needed revision surgery while the other united via secondary bone healing. In this particular study several surgeons, of varied seniority, were the lead surgeon. Both cases were attributed to inadequate screw length, which the investigators believed highlighted the steep learning curve associated with this complex technique.

Surgical-site infections have also been reported in the postoperative period. Rates as high as 5.7% have been published.[51] Very few reports of deep infections have been published, and most settle with the appropriate oral antibiotic therapy. Hammel and colleagues[62] published a 0.8% infection rate in 475 feet. Their main late complication, however, was first MTPJ stiffness. There was a strong declination of stiffness with postoperative time (41.7% at day 35, 5.7% at day 120, 1.3% at 1 year).

Recurrence of the hallux valgus deformity is a further reported event in 3.6% to 6% of cases (see **Fig. 5**).[46,47] Most cases were corrected with an Akin procedure. However, a subsequent arthrodesis has also been used to eradicate symptoms.[47] Undercorrection/recurrence is a possibility, although iatrogenic hallux varus is also a possible scenario. Garrido and colleagues[53] published data on 37 feet with a complication rate of 19%. One of these cases (3%) exhibited a 4° varus deformity, thought to occur secondary to overtightening of the medial capsulorrhaphy. The patient declined surgical correction.

Other complications are rare. Deep vein thrombosis has been reported in 0.6% of cases by Hammel and colleagues.[62] Chronic regional pain syndrome is a documented complication, but controversy exists regarding its prevalence. It has been reported to range between 0% and 4%.[63]

Despite the range of complications, there is an ever-growing body of evidence highlighting the scarf osteotomy as a safe, reliable, and robust technique for hallux valgus

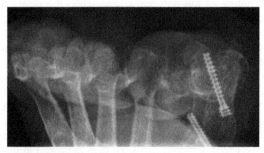

Fig. 5. Sesamoid tunnel view showing long distal screw.

correction. However, as in all surgery, due care must be taken to minimize the risk of a poor outcome.

SUMMARY

The scarf osteotomy is an powerful and versatile method of correcting hallux valgus. It can be used to correct a large range of deformities, including an altered DMAA. As with all operations, complications may arise, but the rate can be diminished by accurate preoperative planning and osteotomy technique.

REFERENCES

1. Barnicot NA, Hardy RH. The position of the hallux in West Africans. J Anat 1955; 89:355–61.
2. MacLennan R. Prevalence of hallux valgus in neolithic New Guinea population. Lancet 1966;1:1398–400.
3. Sim-Fook L, Hodgson AR. A comparison of foot forms among the non-shoe and shoe-wearing Chinese population. J Bone Joint Surg Am 1958;40:1058–62.
4. Kato T, Watanabe S. The etiology of hallux valgus in Japan. Clin Orthop Relat Res 1981;157:78–81.
5. Corrigan JP, Moore DP, Stephens MM. Effect of heel height on forefoot loading. Foot Ankle 1993;14:148–52.
6. Hughes J, Clark P, Jagoe RR, et al. The pattern of pressure distribution under the weight bearing forefoot. Foot 1991;1:117–24.
7. Greer WS. Clinical aspect: relation to footwear. Lancet 1938;232:1482–3.
8. Frey C, Zamora J. The effects of obesity on orthopaedic foot and ankle pathology. Foot Ankle Int 2007;28:996–9.
9. Coughlin MJ, Jones CP. Hallux valgus: demographics, etiology, and radiographic assessment. Foot Ankle Int 2007;28:759–77.
10. Hung LK, Ho YF, Leung PC. Survey of foot deformities among 166 geriatric inpatients. Foot Ankle 1985;5:156–64.
11. Pique-Vidal C, Sole MT, Antich J. Hallux valgus inheritance: pedigree research in 350 patients with bunion deformity. J Foot Ankle Surg 2007;46:149–54.
12. Glynn MK, Dunlop JB, Fitzpatrick D. The Mitchell distal metatarsal osteotomy for hallux valgus. J Bone Joint Surg Br 1980;62-B:188–91.
13. Saro C, Andre B, Wildemyr Z, et al. Outcome after distal metatarsal osteotomy for hallux valgus: a prospective randomized controlled trial of two methods. Foot Ankle Int 2007;28:778–87.
14. Thordarson D, Ebramzadeh E, Moorthy M, et al. Correlation of hallux valgus surgical outcome with AOFAS forefoot score and radiological parameters. Foot Ankle Int 2005;26:122–7.
15. Wilkerson RD, Mason MA. Differences in men's and women's mean ankle ligamentous laxity. Iowa Orthop J 2000;20:46–8.
16. Coughlin MJ, Shurnas PS. Hallux valgus in men. Part II: first ray mobility after bunionectomy and factors associated with hallux valgus deformity. Foot Ankle Int 2003;24:73–8.
17. Frey C, Thompson F, Smith J, et al. American Orthopaedic Foot and Ankle Society women's shoe survey. Foot Ankle 1993;14:78–81.
18. Shine IB. Incidence of hallux valgus in a partially shoe-wearing community. Br Med J 1965;1:1648–50.
19. Robinson AH, Limbers JP. Modern concepts in the treatment of hallux valgus. J Bone Joint Surg Br 2005;87-B:1038–45.

20. Greenberg GS. Relationship of hallux abductus angle and first metatarsal angle to severity of pronation. J Am Podiatry Assoc 1979;69:29–34.

21. Coughlin MJ. Juvenile hallux valgus: etiology and treatment. Foot Ankle Int 1995;16:682–97.

22. Myerson MS, Badekas A. Hypermobility of the first ray. Foot Ankle Clin 2000;5: 469–84.

23. Klaue K, Hansen ST, Masquelet AC. Clinical, quantitative assessment of first tarsometatarsal mobility in the sagittal plane and its relation to hallux valgus deformity. Foot Ankle Int 1994;15:9–13.

24. Lee KT, Young K. Measurement of first-ray mobility in normal vs. hallux valgus patients. Foot Ankle Int 2001;22:960–4.

25. Coughlin MJ, Jones CP, Viladot R, et al. Hallux valgus and first ray mobility: a cadaveric study. Foot Ankle Int 2004;25:537–44.

26. Dreeben S, Mann RA. Advanced hallux valgus deformity: long-term results utilizing the distal soft tissue procedure and proximal metatarsal osteotomy. Foot Ankle Int 1996;17:142–4.

27. Glasoe WM, Allen MK, Ludewig PM. Comparison of first ray dorsal mobility among different forefoot alignments. J Orthop Sports Phys Ther 2000;30:612–20.

28. Tanaka Y, Takakura Y, Kumai T, et al. Radiographic analysis of hallux valgus. A two-dimensional coordinate system. J Bone Joint Surg Am 1995;77:205–13.

29. Perera AM, Mason L, Stephens MM. The pathogenesis of hallux valgus. J Bone Joint Surg Am 2011;93:1650–1.

30. Rush SM, Christensen JC, Johnson CH. Biomechanics of the first ray: part II: metatarsus primus varus as a cause of hypermobility. A three-dimensional kinematic analysis in a cadaver model. J Foot Ankle Surg 2000;39:68–77.

31. Eustace S, Williamson D, Wilson M, et al. Tendon shift in hallux valgus: observations at MR imaging. Skeletal Radiol 1996;25:519–24.

32. Stephens MM. Pathogenesis of hallux valgus. Eur J Foot Ankle Surg 1994;1: 7–10.

33. Wilson DW. Treatment of hallux valgus and bunions. Br J Hosp Med 1980;24: 548–9.

34. Haines RW, McDougall A. The anatomy of hallux valgus. J Bone Joint Surg Br 1954;36:272–93.

35. McBride ED. A conservative operation for bunions. J Bone Joint Surg Am 1928; 10:735–9.

36. Burutaran JM. Hallux valgus y cortedad anatomica del primer metatarsano (correction quirurgica). Actual Med Chir Pied 1976;XIII:261–6.

37. Zygmunt KH, Gudas CJ, Laros GS. Bunionectomy with internal screw fixation. J Am Podiatr Med Assoc 1989;79:322–9.

38. Borrelli AH, Weil LS. Modified scarf bunionectomy: our experience in more than 1000 cases. J Foot Surg 1991;30:609–12.

39. Weil LS. Scarf osteotomy for correction of hallux valgus. Historical perspective, surgical technique and results. Foot Ankle Clin 2000;5:559–80.

40. Barouk LS. Scarf osteotomy of the first metatarsal in the treatment of hallux valgus. Foot Dis 1991;2:35–48.

41. Barouk LS. Scarf osteotomy for hallux valgus correction. Local anatomy, surgical technique, and combination with other forefoot procedures. Foot Ankle Clin 2000;5:525–58.

42. Selvan D, Molloy AP, Abdelmalek A, et al. The effect of preoperative foot and ankle physiotherapy group on reducing inpatient stay and improving patient care. Foot Ankle Surg 2013;19(2):118–20.

43. Holland P, Molloy AP. Intra-operative radiography of scarf osteotomies for hallux valgus. BOFAS Annual Meeting. Newport, November 14–16, 2012.

44. Torkki M, Malmivaara A, Seitsalo S, et al. Surgery vs orthosis vs watchful waiting for hallux valgus: a randomized controlled trial. JAMA 2001;285(19):2474–80.

45. Kitaoka HB, Alexander IJ, Adelaar RS, et al. Clinical rating systems for the ankle-hindfoot, midfoot, hallux, and lesser toes. Foot Ankle Int 1994;15:349–53.

46. Lipscombe S, Molloy A, Sirikonda S, et al. Scarf osteotomy for the correction of hallux valgus: midterm clinical outcome. J Foot Ankle Surg 2008;47(4):273–7.

47. Crevoisier X, Mouhsine E, Ortolano V, et al. The Scarf osteotomy for the treatment of hallux valgus deformity: a review of 84 cases. Foot Ankle Int 2001;22: 970–6.

48. Hardy RH, Clapham JC. Hallux valgus; predisposing anatomical causes. Lancet 1952;1:1180–3.

49. Kristen KH, Berger C, Stelzig S, et al. The SCARF osteotomy for the correction of hallux valgus deformities. Foot Ankle Int 2002;23:221–9.

50. Lorei TJ, Kinast C, Klarner H, et al. Pedographic, clinical, and functional outcome after scarf osteotomy. Clin Orthop Relat Res 2006;451:161–6.

51. Jones S, Al Hussainy HA, Ali F, et al. Scarf osteotomy for hallux valgus. A prospective clinical and pedobarographic study. J Bone Joint Surg Br 2004;86: 830–6.

52. Betts RP, Frank CI, Duckworth T. Foot pressure studies: normal and pathological gait analysis. In: Jahss MH, editor. Disorders of the foot and ankle: medical and surgical management, vol. 1, 2nd edition. Philadelphia: WB Saunders; 1991. p. 484–579.

53. Garrido IM, Rubio ER, Bosch MN, et al. Scarf and Akin osteotomies for moderate and severe hallux valgus: clinical and radiographic results. Foot Ankle Surg 2008;14:194–203.

54. Kerr H, Jackson R, Kothari P. Scarf-Akin osteotomy correction for hallux valgus: short-term results from a district general hospital. J Foot Ankle Surg 2010;49(1): 16–9.

55. Perugia D, Basile A, Gensini A, et al. The scarf osteotomy for severe hallux valgus. Int Orthop 2003;27:103–6.

56. Skotak M, Behounek J. Scarf osteotomy for the treatment of forefoot deformity. Acta Chir Orthop Traumatol Cech 2006;73:18–22.

57. Freslon M, Gayet LE, Bouche G, et al. Scarf osteotomy for the treatment of hallux valgus: a review of 123 cases with 4.8 years follow-up. Rev Chir Orthop Reparatrice Appar Mot 2005;91:257–66.

58. George HL, Casaletto J, Unnikrishnan PN, et al. Outcome of the scarf osteotomy in adolescent hallux valgus. J Child Orthop 2009;3:185–90.

59. Smith S, Landorf K, Butterworth P, et al. Scarf versus chevron osteotomy for the correction of 1-2 intermetatsarsal angle in halux valgus; a systematic review and meta-analysis. J Foot Ankle Surg 2012;51:437–44.

60. Dhukaram V, Hullin MG, Senthil Kumar C. The Mitchell and Scarf osteotomies for hallux valgus correction: a retrospective, comparative analysis using plantar pressures. J Foot Ankle Surg 2006;45:400–9.

61. Desmarchelier R, Besse JL, Fessy MH. Scarf osteotomy versus metatarsophalangeal arthrodesis in forefoot first ray disorders: comparison of functional outcomes. Orthop Traumatol Surg Res 2012;98(Suppl 6):S77–84.

62. Hammel E, Abi Chala ML, Wagner T. Complications of first ray osteotomies: a consecutive series of 475 feet with first metatarsal Scarf osteotomy and first phalanx osteotomy. Rev Chir Orthop Reparatrice Appar Mot 2007;93:710–9.

63. Deenik A, van Mameren H, de Visser E, et al. Equivalent correction in scarf and chevron osteotomy in moderate and severe hallux valgus: a randomized controlled trial. Foot Ankle Int 2008;29:1209–15.

64. Smith AM, Alwan T, Davies MS. Perioperative complications of the scarf osteotomy. Foot Ankle Int 2003;24:222–7.

65. Coetzee JC. Scarf osteotomy for hallux valgus repair: the dark side. Foot Ankle Int 2003;24:29–33.

Minimally Invasive Osteotomies

David Redfern, FRCS(Tr&Orth)[a],*, Anthony Michael Perera, FRCS(Orth)[a,b]

KEYWORDS

- Hallux valgus • Bunion • Minimally invasive • Percutaneous • MICA • Chevron

KEY POINTS

- Specific cadaveric training is mandatory for any surgeon considering performing minimally invasive surgical techniques.
- Cadaveric training is absolutely vital in avoiding unnecessary complications and minimizing the surgeon's learning curve.
- Available data suggest that the minimally invasive Chevron-Akin procedure is a safe alternative to open techniques for hallux valgus correction, although whether minimally invasive techniques such as this offer significant advantages for patients in terms of postoperative morbidity, reduction of stiffness, return to function, and outcome requires further scientific scrutiny.
- Minimally invasive surgical techniques for correction of a wide variety of forefoot and hindfoot abnormalities are currently gaining popularity among European surgeons, and this is an interesting area of development.

INTRODUCTION

During the past 20 years, surgery has seen an inexorable trend toward less invasive and keyhole approaches. For instance, in the field of general surgery, laparoscopic cholecystectomy and appendicectomy have become firmly established as the surgical gold standards. If an equivalent technical result to an open surgical procedure is possible to achieve with a safe but less invasive approach, then better patient outcomes ought to follow, and the profession should continue to strive in this direction.

Orthopedics has not been left behind in this less invasive evolution. Arthroscopic ankle cheilectomy and arthroscopic ankle fusion are replacing open approaches. However, minimally invasive hallux valgus surgery has been slower to establish. In fact, the number of proposed open procedures to treat this condition continues to increase. However, the Arbeitsgemeinschaft für Osteosynthesefragen (AO) group's principles of minimizing soft tissue trauma and periosteal stripping are just as relevant to hallux valgus surgery as they are to fracture management.

[a] London Foot & Ankle Centre, Hospital St John & St Elizabeth, 60 Grove End Road, London NW8 9NH, UK; [b] Spire Cardiff Hospital, Croescadarn Road, Cardiff, CF23 8XL, UK
* Corresponding author.
E-mail address: davidjredfern@me.com

Foot Ankle Clin N Am 19 (2014) 181–189
http://dx.doi.org/10.1016/j.fcl.2014.02.002
1083-7515/14/$ – see front matter © 2014 Elsevier Inc. All rights reserved.

Perhaps this reluctance to embrace minimally invasive techniques in hallux valgus correction is partly explained by the general perception that bunions are "easy to do and easy to get wrong."

In fact, a literature review shows that approximately 85% of patients report good outcome after open hallux valgus correction. Analysis of the remaining 15% reveals frequent issues with stiffness and pain related to the soft tissues rather than purely osteotomy issues. Thus, perhaps the key to improving outcome after hallux valgus surgery lies in a less invasive soft tissue approach rather than which of the myriad described osteotomies is used. That said, early minimally invasive techniques failed to adhere to the AO principles of rigid internal fixation and early mobilization and have been associated with poor outcomes, adding fuel to concerns that "minimally invasive" equates to "easier to get it wrong."

PRINCIPLES OF MINIMALLY INVASIVE SURGERY

The term *minimally invasive* refers to the skin incision/approach, not the type of osteotomy used. Despite this, several disparate operations using minimally invasive techniques are frequently grouped together under the "minimally invasive" banner in a way that does not make sense and does not occur when referring to open techniques. The ability to differentiate between different techniques is important for meaningful and rational comparison to be made.

EVOLUTION OF MINIMALLY INVASIVE FIRST METATARSAL OSTEOTOMIES

Less invasive procedures were promoted by Wilson[1] and Bösch and colleagues[2] in the 1980s. The latter was a more percutaneous approach and used a subcapital Hohmann osteotomy[3] through a short vertical incision at the level of the neck of the metatarsal. However, the first truly minimally invasive technique to gain prominence was a modification of the Reverdin osteotomy[4] developed by Stephen Isham[5] published in 1985 (and more recently popularized by Mariano De Prado in Spain).[6] Isham[5] developed a modification of the Shannon burr with end and side cutting performance to perform an oblique medial closing wedge osteotomy of the head of the first metatarsal. The osteotomy was extra-articular but intracapsular. He combined this with a minimally invasive Akin operation, bunionectomy, and adductor release. He believed that this construct was sufficiently stable that no internal fixation was required, and used postoperative rehabilitation as for a minimal incision Silver-Akin procedure, using postoperative splint dressings to stabilize the correction.

Isham and Nunez[7] stated that a marked improvement of short-term and long-term results were immediately apparent. However, although these investigators acknowledge that the average shortening is 5 mm and that this can be greater, they do not describe any related complications.

The lack of fixation and the degree of shortening inherent in this procedure are causes for concern, and the results have not been reproduced[8] despite the large-scale uptake by podiatrists in the United States in the 1970s to 1990s. In fact, sparse independent literature exists on the Reverdin-Isham procedure.

Perhaps because of poor experiences associated with these early minimally invasive techniques,[9] little interest has been shown in minimally invasive surgery in the United States in recent years. The next stage of development has occurred in Europe, where several centers have been developing minimally invasive techniques and showing positive results with reduced inpatient stay and better recovery,[10] which has served to reignite interest and add momentum to the evolution.

The Bosch osteotomy has regained interest in Europe and was popularized by Magnan and colleagues[11,12] and Giannini and colleagues,[13] who called his modification the *SERI* (Simple, Effective, Rapid, Inexpensive). Excellent results with full correction, mean American Orthopaedic Foot & Ankle Society (AOFAS) scores of 91.8, and no significant complications have been published,[14] even at 10-year follow-up.[15] However, it is concerning that these procedures use an inherently unstable vertical osteotomy at the level of the neck, which is splinted by a single K-wire (passed through the soft-tissues of the medial hallux and then run down the medullary canal of the metatarsal) rather than rigidly internally fixed.

Independent analyses of this technique have generally failed to reproduce good results,[16] even with a second K-wire to transfix the osteotomy.[17] In a prospective study, Kadakia and colleagues[9] reported almost universally poor results even at short-term follow-up, with some patients experiencing major complications, such as dorsal malunion (70%), recurrence (40%), osteonecrosis, and wound complications. The investigators discontinued the study after only 3 months because of the magnitude and frequency of the complications observed.

MINIMALLY INVASIVE CHEVRON-AKIN

The wish to pursue the sound (AO) principles of modern fracture fixation must lead not only in the direction of less invasive (or perhaps better described as less disruptive) soft tissue surgery but also toward stable internal fracture fixation. Thus, applying this to hallux valgus surgery, the objective should be to achieve an accurate and controllable osteotomy with stable internal fixation without compromising the soft tissue envelope of the fracture or adjacent hallux metatarsophalangeal joint (MTPJ). It is from these objectives that the minimally invasive Chevron-Akin (MICA) has been proposed. Developed by Joel Vernois and David Redfern in the United Kingdom,[18] this technique involves the use of percutaneous surgical techniques to create a chevron-type osteotomy at the level of the distal diaphyseal-metaphyseal junction of the first metatarsal and an Akin-type osteotomy of the hallux proximal phalanx, both of which are internally fixed with compression screws and combined with a percutaneous distal soft tissue release.

The MICA technique is the first minimally invasive hallux valgus correction technique to truly marry the perceived advantages of an extracapsular first metatarsal osteotomy in which the fracture soft tissue envelope is preserved with rigid internal fixation.

MICA SURGICAL TECHNIQUE

The MICA procedure can be performed under general anesthesia and/or ankle block and no tourniquet is required, although this author (D.R.) prefers to use one. The patient is positioned supine with the feet overhanging the end of the operating table to facilitate intraoperative imaging in any plane with a mini C-arm.

Using a beaver blade, a 3-mm incision is made on the dorsomedial border of the first metatarsal at the base of the flare of the medial eminence (distal diaphyseal-metaphyseal junction). Through this incision, a specific straight periosteal elevator is used to create a puncture in the medial capsule over the apex of the medial eminence (ie, introduced subcutaneously in a distal direction, entering the first MTPJ just distal to the capsular attachment on the medial eminence). Then a 3.1-mm wedge burr is used to remove the distal medial eminence, preserving the proximal eminence, which is required later to displace the chevron osteotomy (**Fig. 1**). The chevron osteotomy is then created using a Shannon burr of 2-mm diameter and 20-mm length. The burr is introduced via the same initial skin incision at the level of the neck of the metatarsal.

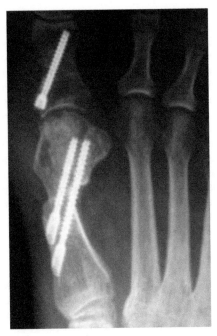

Fig. 1. Removal of the distal bunion eminence.

The orientation of the burr is particularly important when initially introducing it through the first metatarsal. This first plunge of the burr will become the apex of chevron and will determine the subsequent displacement of the osteotomy in all 3 planes and hence the final correction. It is important to remember that the burr is 2 mm in diameter and will cut a channel in the bone of 2- to 3-mm diameter. Thus, if the burr is introduced perpendicular to the second metatarsal in the transverse plane, this will create shortening of approximately 2 to 3 mm. This effect may be desirable, but if not, the burr should be directed distally by approximately 10° to avoid this shortening. In the same way, if the burr is introduced perpendicular to the second metatarsal in the coronal plane, this will create elevation of approximately 2 mm (**Fig. 2**). This elevation can be avoided by directing the burr in a more plantar direction

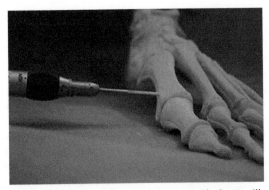

Fig. 2. A cut perpendicular to the second ray in the coronal plane will create elevation of the head fragment from the bone removed by the 2-mm diameter of the burr.

of approximately 10° (if desired, plantarization of the first metatarsal head can be achieved by increasing this angle). With this awareness, the surgeon can accurately plan the required/desired plane of displacement of the osteotomy (**Fig. 3**).

Once the initial plunge of the burr has been performed and hence the plane of the osteotomy set, then the dorsal and plantar limbs of the chevron (V-shaped) osteotomy are completed from this point.

When the osteotomy has been completed, either a 2-mm K-wire (for smaller displacements) or the specific periosteal elevator tool (for larger displacements) is inserted into the osteotomy and the proximal diaphyseal channel. This procedure is performed via either the same initial incision or an additional 3-mm skin incision over the summit of the bunion eminence (which helps to control the instrument). This wire/elevator is then used as a lever to displace the head along the created osteotomy path. The displacement is then checked in both anteroposterior and lateral planes using the image intensifier and adjusted if necessary. The wire/elevator is removed once the osteotomy has been internally fixed with screws.

Stable internal fixation is achieved using 2 specifically designed cannulated compression screws. These screws are introduced via proximal medial stab incisions under image-intensifier guidance. The key to achieving rigid fixation is the need to pass the more proximal of these screws through both cortices of the proximal first metatarsal diaphysis before it enters the displaced metatarsal head fragment, thereby achieving 3-point fixation (**Fig. 4**). The second screw adds to the stability and strength of the construct and controls rotation.

A distal soft tissue release is then performed (not before the chevron osteotomy) using a beaver blade introduced into the lateral recess of the first metatarsophalangeal joint via an additional 3-mm skin incision. The blade is then pushed into the plantar plate and the lateral sesamoid phalangeal ligament (lateral head of flexor hallucis brevis) is divided. Alternatively, the suspensory ligament can be divided using the same approach.

In 50% to 60% of cases, a percutaneous Akin osteotomy of the hallux proximal phalanx is also performed with percutaneous internal screw fixation.

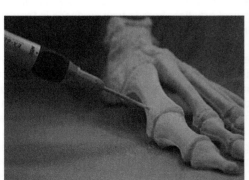
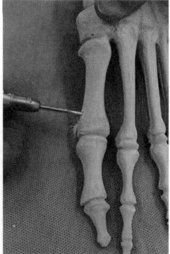

Fig. 3. Correct direction of cut to accommodate for diameter of burr (10° beyond perpendicular to the second ray in both coronal and transverse planes).

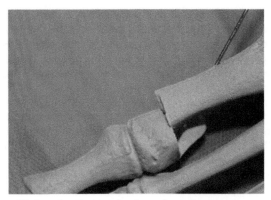

Fig. 4. Sawbone model showing 3-point fixation of proximal screw.

Final clinical inspection and intraoperative radiographs ensure satisfactory correction and fixation (**Fig. 5**A, B).

Postoperatively, the patient is allowed to full weight-bear in a flat postoperative shoe for 5 to 6 weeks. At that stage, they are reviewed with standing anteroposterior and lateral radiographs to confirm maintenance of correction before being allowed to migrate into ordinary footwear.

The authors have extensive experience with this technique (>500 cases) and have observed a very low incidence of postoperative stiffness, such that routine postoperative physiotherapy is not required. Generally, lateral displacements of 80% can easily be achieved, but, with experience, very large deformities can be corrected with 100% displacement of the osteotomy and maintaining stable rigid internal fixation. There seems to be very reliable union, and the authors have not encountered any incidences of nonunion or avascular necrosis to date. Remodeling of the first metatarsal occurs gradually over 4 to 12 months (see **Fig. 5**C).

RESULTS

Use of this technique is increasing in Europe, although few data have been published in terms of results.[18] Vernois[18,19] and Redfern and colleagues,[18,20,21] and Perera[22] have presented their early results with the MICA technique at both the British and American Orthopaedic Foot & Ankle Societies.

As with any new technique, there is a learning curve. Cadaveric courses are mandatory before using this technique in clinical practice, both to train surgeons in the safe use of the burrs and to help them learn the MICA technique itself and how to avoid pitfalls (as with any technique).

In 2010, Redfern and Walker[21] presented early learning curve results for the MICA technique (including technique modifications) performed in 70 patients (83 osteotomies). Satisfactory improvement was seen in both intermetatarsal and hallux valgus angles and Kitaoka scores at 3- to 12-month follow-up. Overall, 94% of patients were satisfied or very satisfied with the results of surgery. In this initial series, only 5 patients (7%) experienced movement of the osteotomy during the early postoperative period (with only 2 patients requiring further corrective surgery). As a result of these cases, the fixation technique was modified (tricortical fixation with proximal screw) to successfully avoid this problem. Transfer metatarsalgia was observed in 4 patients, and 2 superficial wound infections, no deep infections, and no cases of osteonecrosis were seen.

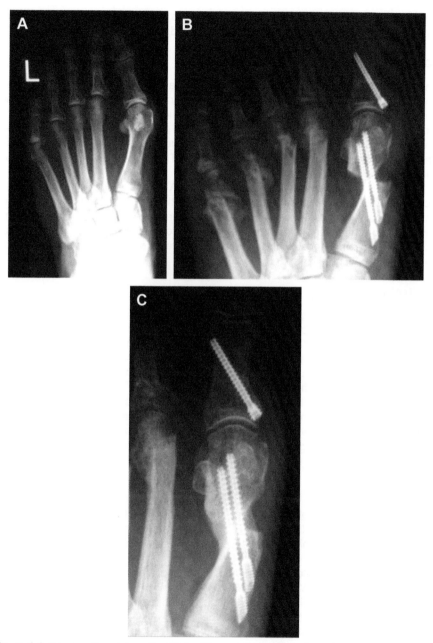

Fig. 5. (*A*) Preoperative deformity. (*B*) Position maintained at 6 weeks postsurgery (note 3-point fixation with proximal screw). (*C*) Remodeling at 4 months postsurgery.

In 2013, Perera presented his early learning curve experience with the MICA technique in a comparative study of the MICA technique versus open chevron osteotomies (AOFAS 2013). These results were also very encouraging. Manchester-Oxford Foot Questionnaire and AOFAS scores were significantly better in the MICA group than the open chevron group. Perera also observed a lower infection rate and less postoperative stiffness and pain in the MICA group than in the open chevron group, with no significant difference in correction achieved.

POTENTIAL COMPLICATIONS

The potential complications of the MICA technique are the same as those of any open hallux valgus technique and those of using a burr percutaneously (eg, portal burn). The authors have not experienced any of these complications with the proposed technique, but without training and awareness of these potential risks, they are possible. The results thus far suggest that the MICA technique may be associated with a lower risk of infection, less stiffness (because the first MTPJ capsule is not violated as it is with open techniques), and less pain.

No reports exist of osteonecrosis with the MICA technique. Beyond this, as with open techniques, the potential risks of undercorrection or overcorrection of the hallux valgus deformity remain and are user- and experience-dependent. Any surgeons wishing to perform the MICA technique must undergo specialist cadaveric training from surgeons experienced with the technique to reduce the learning curve and potential complications.

SUMMARY

Specific cadaveric training is mandatory for any surgeon considering performing minimally invasive surgical techniques. This training is absolutely vital in avoiding unnecessary complications and minimizing the surgeon's learning curve.

Available data suggest that the MICA technique is a safe alternative to open techniques for hallux valgus correction, although whether minimally invasive techniques such as this offer significant advantages for patients in terms of postoperative morbidity, reduction of stiffness, return to function, and outcome requires further scientific scrutiny as surgeons publish their data. Minimally invasive surgical techniques for correction of a wide variety of forefoot and hindfoot abnormalities are currently gaining popularity among European surgeons, and this is an interesting area of development.

REFERENCES

1. Wilson D. Treatment of hallux valgus and bunions. Br J Hosp Med 1980;24:548–9.
2. Bösch P, Wanke S, Legenstein R. Hallux valgus correction by the method of Bösch: a new technique with a seven-to-ten year follow-up. Foot Ankle Clin 2000;5:485–98.
3. Hohmann G. Symptomatische oder physiologische Behandlung des Hallux valgus. Munch Med Wochenschr 1921;68:1042–5.
4. Reverdin J. De la deviation en dehors du gros orl (hallux valgus) et son traitement chirurgical. Trans Int Med Congress 1881;2:408–12.
5. Isham S. The Reverdin-Isham procedure for the correction of hallux abducto valgus. A distal metatarsal osteotomy procedure. Clin Podiatr Med Surg 1991; 8:81–94.
6. De Prado M, Ripoll PL, Golano P, Minimally Invasive Foot Surgery: Surgical Techniques, Indications, Anatomical Basis. Bilbao, Spain: About Your Health. 2009. ISBN 8461316096, 9788461316090.
7. Isham SA, Nunez OE. The Reverdin-Isham procedure for the correction of hallux valgus. In: Maffulli N, Easley M, editors. Minimally invasive surgery of the foot and ankle. London: Springer-Verlag; 2011. p. 97–108.

8. Bauer T, Biau D, Lortat-Jacob A, et al. Percutaneous hallux valgus correction using the Reverdin-Isham osteotomy. Orthop Traumatol Surg Res 2010;96(4): 407–16.
9. Kadakia AR, Smerek JP, Myerson MS. Radiographic results after percutaneous distal metatarsal osteotomy for correction of hallux valgus deformity. Foot Ankle Int 2007;28:355–60.
10. Leemrijse T, Valtin B, Besse JL. Hallux valgus surgery in 2005. Conventional, mini-invasive or percutaneous surgery? Uni- or bilateral? Hospitalisation or one-day surgery? Rev Chir Orthop Reparatrice Appar Mot 2008;94:111–27.
11. Magnan B, Montanari M, Bragantini A, et al. Trattamento chirurgico dell'alluce valgo con tecnica "mini-invasiva" percutanea (P.D.O.: percutaneous distal osteotomy). In: Malerba F, Dragonetti L, Giannini S, editors. Progressi in medicina e chirurgia del piede. Volume 6, L'alluce valgo. Bologna (Italy): Aulo Gaggi; 1997. p. 91–104.
12. Magnan B, Pezzè L, Rossi N, et al. Percutaneous distal metatarsal osteotomy for correction of hallux valgus. J Bone Joint Surg Am 2005;87:1191–9.
13. Giannini S, Ceccarelli F, Bevoni R, et al. Hallux valgus surgery: the minimally invasive bunion correction. Tech Foot Ankle Surg 2003;2:11–20.
14. Tong CK, Ho YF. Use of minimally invasive distal metatarsal osteotomy for correction of hallux valgus. J Orthop Trauma Rehabil 2012;16:16–21.
15. Faour-Martín O, Martín-Ferrero MA, Valverde García JA, et al. Long-term results of the retrocapital metatarsal percutaneous osteotomy for hallux valgus. Int Orthop 2013;37(9):1799–803.
16. Iannò B, Familiari F, De Gori M, et al. Midterm results and complications after minimally invasive distal metatarsal osteotomy for treatment of hallux valgus. Foot Ankle Int 2013;34(7):969–77.
17. Huang PJ, Lin YC, Fu YC, et al. Radiographic evaluation of minimally invasive distal metatarsal osteotomy for hallux valgus. Foot Ankle Int 2011;32(5):S503–7.
18. Vernois J, Redfern DJ. Percutaneous Chevron; the union of classic stable fixed approach and percutaneous technique. Fuss & Sprunggelenk 2013;11(2):70–5.
19. Vernois J. The treatment of the hallux valgus with a percutaneous chevron osteotomy. J Bone Joint Surg Br 2011;93(Suppl IV):482.
20. Redfern D, Gill I, Harris M. Early experience with a minimally invasive modified chevron and akin osteotomy for correction of hallux valgus. J Bone Joint Surg Br 2011;93(Suppl IV):482.
21. Walker R, Redfern D. Experience with a minimally invasive distal lesser metatarsal osteotomy for the treatment of metatarsalgia. J Bone Joint Surg Br 2012; 94(Suppl XXII):39.
22. Perera AM, Beddard L, Marudunayam A. Paper presented at American Orthopaedic Foot and Ankle Society Summer meeting. Hollywood, Fl, July, 2013.

Correction of Moderate and Severe Hallux Valgus Deformity with a Distal Metatarsal Osteotomy Using an Intramedullary Plate

Ezequiel Palmanovich, MD*, Mark S. Myerson, MD

KEYWORD

- Severe hallux valgus • Distal metatarsal osteotomy • Chevron • Correction power
- Intramedullar plate • Novel technique

KEY POINTS

- The concept of minor and moderate deformities being treated by distal osteotomies and the severe deformities treated best by proximal metatarsal osteotomies is changing.
- High, powerful correction for aggressive distal chevron osteotomy can be fixed by a stable intramedullar plate.
- A new technique of fixation is based on the Murawski and Beskin concept, because a powerful correction can be performed with a minimally invasive approach.
- A low rate of complications is due to minimal invasive technique.

INTRODUCTION

Hallux valgus is defined as a subluxation of the first metatarsophalangeal (MP) joint with lateral deviation of the great toe and medial deviation of the first metatarsal.[1] Between 2% and 4% of the population are affected by this deformity[2] and 84% of patients have a positive family history, most commonly from maternal transmission.[3] More than 200 surgeries have been described for hallux valgus correction,[4] including the use of various osteotomies, with good success rates and reliability over time.[5] The distal V-shape chevron-type osteotomy, in the class of distal metatarsal osteotomies, was first described by Corless,[6] Johnson and colleagues,[7] and Austin and Leventen[8] and was typically indicated for correction of mild to moderate deformity.

In these earlier articles, it was recommended that for correction of a distal metatarsal osteotomy approximately 25% but no more than 50% translation of the distal

---

Institute for the Foot and Ankle Reconstruction, Mercy Hospital, 301 St. Paul Place, Baltimore, MD 21202, USA
* Corresponding author.
E-mail address: ezepalm@gmail.com

Foot Ankle Clin N Am 19 (2014) 191–201
http://dx.doi.org/10.1016/j.fcl.2014.02.003
1083-7515/14/$ – see front matter © 2014 Elsevier Inc. All rights reserved.

foot.theclinics.com

fragment in relation to the metatarsal shaft should be attempted.[6–8] Subsequently, Badwey and colleagues[9] in an anatomic study suggested that the capital fragment can be safely shifted 6 mm in men and 5 mm in women while maintaining 50% of bone apposition. Given that the average width of the first metatarsal at the level of the neck is about 12 mm in women and 14 mm in men,[10] the recommendations of Badwey and Corless are quite similar. However, correction with this type of osteotomy is limited by the amount of lateral translation that can safely be performed, because the risk of instability, delayed union, and malunion potentially increase with greater shifts of the metatarsal head.[11–13] In conjunction with the amount of shift of the distal metatarsal that could be performed, it was recognized that there was a similar limit to the correction of the intermetatarsal (IM) deformity with this and other distal metatarsal osteotomies. Recommendations for these distally based osteotomy procedures have therefore been described by many authors, limiting the correction to an IM angle less than 14°.[13–21] In general, therefore, more severe deformities have been best treated by proximal metatarsal osteotomies; these have been proven mathematically as well as clinically to give the more predictable correction than the distal metatarsal osteotomy regardless of type.[4,5,22,23] However, these proximal osteotomies have a higher complication rate, a higher rate of recurrence, and a greater morbidity for the patient postoperatively. They typically require longer periods of immobilization, at times with no weight-bearing permitted. Therefore, there would be a distinct advantage if a distal metatarsal osteotomy could be performed for greater or more severe deformities.

Various reports attest to the possibility of using a distal metatarsal osteotomy to correct greater deformity.[10,24–27] However, these procedures have been performed with inherently unstable forms of fixation. The Kramer procedure consists of an open technique with a distal lateral translational osteotomy and fixed by a k-wire that is placed in medial soft tissue of the proximal phalanx and passed across the MP joint into the intramedullary canal, simultaneously pushing the metatarsal head laterally. The percutaneous Bosch[25] technique is very similar but the osteotomy is performed by perforating the subcapital cortex of the metatarsal and manually breaking; the fixation is similar. In the Giannini[26] technique, the minimally invasive transverse metatarsal neck osteotomy is performed using a saw and fixed in a similar way. Magnan and colleagues[10] used the micromotorized Linderman bone cutter for the osteotomy. Although the mean IM angle in the study of Bosch and colleagues[25] improved from 13 to 10° and Magnan and colleagues[10] from 12 to 7°, the reported results of these procedures have been fair with numerous complications, particularly malunion and stiffness of the MP joint. In a later similar study of a minimally invasive distal metatarsal osteotomy with percutaneous pin fixation by Kadakia and colleagues,[27] these procedures were all noted to have a very high rate of complications, largely because of the method of fixation and the inherent instability of the osteotomy as well as the transarticular fixation. There have been no long-term published studies of distal metatarsal osteotomy with a minimally invasive technique using traditional methods of internal fixation.

However, the possibility of using a distally based osteotomy for correction of more severe deformity was pursued by Murawski and Beskin,[28] who modified the distal chevron osteotomy procedure. They recommended performing the procedure with the apex of the osteotomy 15 to 20 mm proximal to the articular surface and the limbs made more acutely at an angle of 35 to 45°, exiting the diaphysis of the metatarsal. They noted that if the limbs of the osteotomy are too short, there may be excessive instability, but when cut too long, there may be difficulty translating or rotating the distal head portion. The osteotomy is completed with a sagittal saw and the distal head fragment is gently translated laterally while applying traction to the toe. The head fragment is perched on the lateral spike of the proximal fragment, and Murawski and Beskin noted that up to 90% translation is possible and satisfactorily stabilized with one or two 0.054-inch smooth Kirschner wires. Kirschner wires are placed percutaneously from the medial aspect of the proximal fragment, across the osteotomy site, and into the head fragment. The large prominence of bone from the more proximal medial metatarsal diaphysis is cut and contoured in line with the distal head at the medial margin.

The results of the technique reported by Murawski and Beskin were encouraging and prompted the authors to investigate the ability to correct moderate to severe deformity with a distally based metatarsal osteotomy. More recently, a new method of intramedullary fixation for correction of the distal metatarsal osteotomy has been made available (Orthohelix Mini MaxLock Extreme ISO). This plate permits significant shift of the distal metatarsal but provides inherent stability to the osteotomy.

SURGICAL TECHNIQUE

An incision is made medially at the junction of the dorsal and plantar skin, extending proximally for 3 cm from the MP joint. The soft tissues are dissected carefully to identify the terminal medial cutaneous branch of the superficial peroneal nerve. Depending on the approach taken, the procedure can be performed following a traditional capsulotomy with a chevron-type cut in the metatarsal neck, or a more proximally based osteotomy that does not need to be intracapsular. The osteotomy may be either chevron-shaped or transverse, depending on the magnitude of correction required and the orientation of the osteotomy (**Fig. 1**). The authors prefer to use the straight osteotomy and not the chevron cut when the deformity is greater (ie, greater

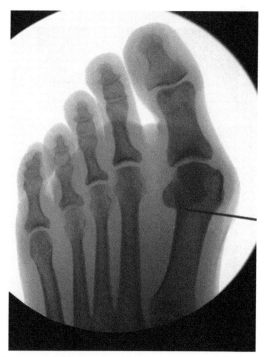

Fig. 1. Surgical technique: cut landmark.

than 15°). It is more versatile and can be inclined so as to translate the metatarsal in a plantar and proximal direction if necessary. If the procedure is intracapsular, then a horizontally oriented capsular incision is placed slightly more toward the plantar aspect of the metatarsal head. It is not necessary to perform a medial exostectomy with either technique because the metatarsal head is shifted far laterally and is not at all prominent. The advantage of the chevron cut here is (as noted by Murawski and Beskin) the potential for a greater surface area of the osteotomy; however, this may not provide any more stability than a horizontal osteotomy cut with the fixation used in the authors series.

Multiplanar correction is possible by orientating the saw blade slightly proximal or toward the plantar. On completion of the osteotomy, it is distracted and the metatarsal head is then pushed over laterally manually while the metatarsal shaft is held stable (**Fig. 2**). A small k-wire can be inserted through the metatarsal head to achieve temporary stability. Once the desired shift is achieved, the broach is placed against the flat surface of the metatarsal head. The broach determines placement and orientation of the plate, which is then inserted into the intramedullary canal (**Fig. 3**). Once the plate is properly positioned, a 1.6-mm drill bit is performed for the 2.4-mm locking screws in the metatarsal head. It is important to ensure that the orientation of the plate is correct on the medial surface of the metatarsal head and not rotated to its dorsomedial surface. Once the plate is secure to the metatarsal head, a lag screw is inserted into the pocket of the plate, which locks the lateral proximal cortex of the first metatarsal, thereby providing compression and stability to the system (**Fig. 4**).

The plate can be inserted either parallel with the lateral cortex of the first metatarsal or at an angle, depending on the desired orientation of the metatarsal head. If, for example, an increase of the distal metatarsal articular angle is present, then the plate can be inserted into the metatarsal at a slight angle (ie, aimed slightly medially with

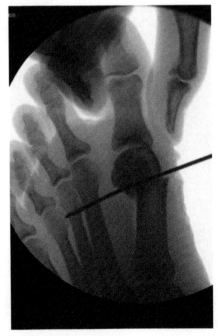

Fig. 2. Surgical technique: transverse osteotomy.

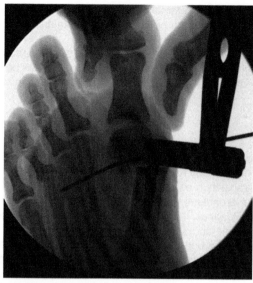

Fig. 3. Surgical technique: intramedullar plate insertion.

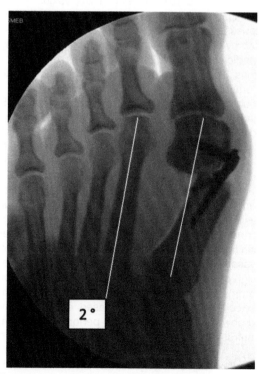

Fig. 4. Surgical technique: intramedullar plate fixation and final IM angle measurement.

reference to the axis of the metatarsal), and this will reorientate the distal metatarsal articular angle into a more neutral position as the metatarsal head is affixed to the plate.

If necessary, a percutaneous soft tissue release is now performed with a small Beaver Blade. It is not recommended that a soft tissue release be performed before the osteotomy, because this will add to instability of the head when translating it laterally.

DISCUSSION

The first to describe distal osteotomy was Barker[29] in 1884 with a distal closing wedge, which was modified by Kramer,[24,30] who replaced the closing wedge osteotomy with a lateral translation osteotomy and Kirschner wire fixation. The results of this modified Kramer technique were compared with the Austin or Chevron osteotomy by Trnka and colleagues,[31] showing that the Kramer technique was associated with more malalignment and recurrent hallux valgus deformity. Bosch and colleagues[25] simplified this procedure further by developing an osteotomy that was fixed by a novel technique of insertion of the Kirschner wire through the first MP joint medial capsule. However, a significant limitation of this approach is that the surgeon is unable to control the magnitude of lateral translation, and the osteotomy is not stable with this type of fixation; because of the transarticular fixation, joint stiffness is likely.[5,32]

These same criticisms apply to the invasive SERI osteotomy (simple, effective, rapid, and inexpensive) described by Giannini and colleagues.[26] They reported no complications in a series of 40 patients with hallux valgus,[32] which is in marked contrast to the investigation by Kadakia and colleagues[27] and by Fernández de Retana and colleagues.[33] In the latter study, the SERI technique was compared with the scarf osteotomy (SCARF) in 40 patients, finding significantly more complication, including 2 superficial infections, 2 deep infections, 6 cases of hardware intolerance, 3 delayed unions, 3 cases of complete metatarsal head displacement, 12 cases of first metatarsal dorsal displacement, and 23 undercorrections.

Special credit should be given to the procedure written by James Beskin and Daniel Murawski,[28] a modification of the technique as originally described by Corless,[6] Austin and Leventen,[8] and Johnson and colleagues.[7] In their technique, head fragment is translated laterally with up to 90% translation and satisfactorily stabilized with two 0.054-inch smooth Kirschner wires. Badwey and colleagues[9] reported that the capital fragment can be displaced laterally up to 6 mm in men and 5 mm in women, which constitutes displacement of approximately 30% of the metatarsal's width. However, Murawski and Beskin[28] concluded after 2 years of follow-up of 62 patients and 72 procedures that increasing the displacement of distal chevron osteotomy can provide more powerful deformity correction and can be applied to a broader range of preoperative deformity than traditional techniques without increased risk of malunion, recurrence, nonunion, avascular necrosis, or transfer lesions.

This concept of high powerful correction for distal chevron osteotomy fixed by the Mini MaxLock Extreme ISO gives the surgeon the possibility of a mini-invasive rapid solution. This new technique of fixation is based on the Murawski and Beskin concept, because a powerful correction can be performed with a minimally invasive approach, but in contrast to other studies discussed above, with stable osteotomy fixation (Figs. 5–7).

Complications of hallux valgus surgery depend on inherent stability of the osteotomy, the type of fixation, and the anatomic location of the osteotomy.[34–36] The

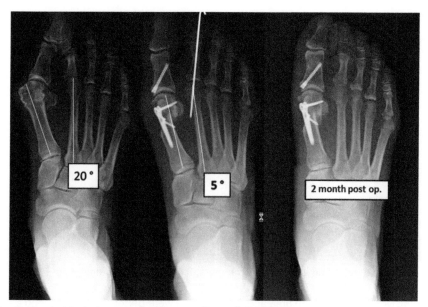

Fig. 5. Surgical technique: pre- and postradiograph IM angle measurement.

complications associated with the traditional distal chevron osteotomy include recurrent hallux valgus, overcorrection resulting in varus deformity, and avascular necrosis.[37] In the authors' series of the first 25 patients, 2 cases were found. The first case was a nonunion case that was a complaint of local pain. In the radiograph 9 months after surgery, an obvious nonunion at the site of the osteotomy was found

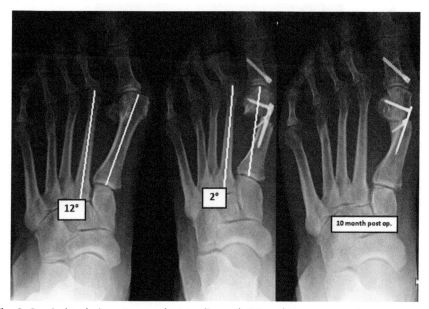

Fig. 6. Surgical technique: pre- and postradiograph IM angle measurement.

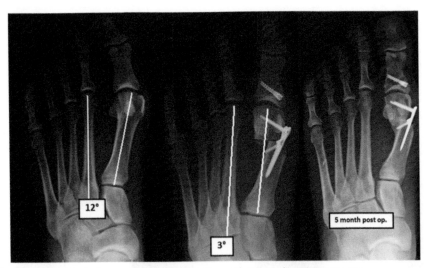

Fig. 7. Surgical technique: pre- and postradiograph IM angle measurement.

(**Fig. 8**). Debridement of the area and bone grafting were performed. The second case had excellent correction initially but deformity recurred because of TMT instability and a Lapidus procedure was performed (**Fig. 9**). There are 2 more cases of superficial wound infection treated with oral antibiotics and resolved without further complications.

The technique of fixation introduced here has taken into consideration all different variants of deformity to decrease the complication rate, displacement, correction, stability, and fixation for the distal metatarsal osteotomy.

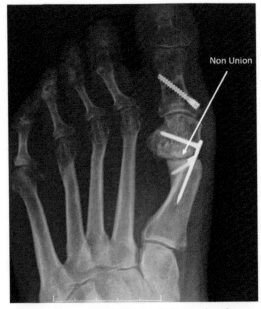

Fig. 8. Nonunion at the osteotomy site. Radiograph 9 months after surgery.

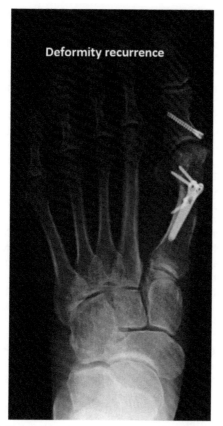

Fig. 9. Recurrence of deformity due to tarso metatarsal instability.

SUMMARY

The historical concept of minor and moderate deformities being treated by distal osteotomies and the severe deformities treated best by proximal metatarsal osteotomies is now changing with this new intramedullary plate fixation for distal chevron osteotomies. Correction of severe deformation can be corrected with aggressive chevron osteotomy and stable intramedullar plate fixation.

REFERENCES

1. Smith BW, Coughlin MJ. Treatment of hallux valgus with increased distal metatarsal articular angle: use of double and triple osteotomies. Foot Ankle Clin 2009;14(3):369.
2. Myerson MS. Foot and ankle disorders, hallux valgus. Philadelphia: WB Saunders; 1999. p. 213.
3. Coughlin MJ, Jones CP. Hallux valgus: demographics, etiology, and radiographic assessment. Foot Ankle Int 2007;28:759.
4. Wagner E, Ortiz C. Osteotomy considerations in hallux valgus treatment: improving the correction power. Foot Ankle Clin 2012;17(3):481.
5. Trnka HJ. Osteotomies for hallux valgus correction. Foot Ankle Clin 2005;10:15.

6. Corless JR. A modification of the Mitchell procedure. J Bone Joint Surg Br 1976; 55:138.
7. Johnson KA, Cofield RH, Morrey BF. Chevron osteotomy for hallux valgus. Clin Orthop 1979;142:44.
8. Austin DW, Leventen EO. A new osteotomy for hallux valgus: a horizontally directed "V" displacement osteotomy of the metatarsal head for hallux valgus and primus varus. Clin Orthop Relat Res 1981;(157):25.
9. Badwey TM, Dutkowsky JP, Graves SC, et al. An anatomical basis for the degree of displacement of the distal chevron osteotomy in the treatment of hallux valgus. Foot Ankle Int 1997;18:213.
10. Jahss MH, Troy AI, Kummer F. Roentgenographic and mathematical analysis of first metatarsal osteotomies for metatarsus primus varus: a comparative study. Foot Ankle 1985;5(6):280–321.
11. Hattrup SJ, Johnson KA. Chevron osteotomy: analysis of factors of patients' dissatisfaction. Foot Ankle Int 1985;5:327.
12. Mann RA, Coughlin MJ. Adult hallux valgus. In: Coughlin MJ, Mann RA, editors. Surgery of the foot and ankle. 7th edition. St Louis (MO): Mosby; 1999. p. 150.
13. Meier PJ, Kenzora JE. The risks and benefits of distal first metatarsal osteotomies. Foot Ankle Int 1985;6:7.
14. Caminear DS, Pavlovich R Jr, Pietrzak WS. Fixation of the chevron osteotomy with an absorbable copolymer pin for treatment of hallux valgus deformity. J Foot Ankle Surg 2005;44(3):203.
15. Chen YJ, Hsu RW, Shih HN, et al. Distal chevron osteotomy with intra-articular lateral soft-tissue release for treatment of moderate to severe hallux valgus deformity. J Formos Med Assoc 1996;95(10):776.
16. Crosby LA, Bozarth GR. Fixation comparison for chevron osteotomies. Foot Ankle Int 1998;19(1):41.
17. Mann RA, Donatto KC. The chevron osteotomy: a clinical and radiographic analysis. Foot Ankle Int 1997;18(5):255.
18. Peterson DA, Zilberfarb JL, Greene MA, et al. Avascular necrosis of the first metatarsal head: incidence in distal osteotomy combined with lateral soft tissue release. Foot Ankle Int 1994;15(2):59.
19. Pochatko DJ, Schlehr FJ, Murphey MD, et al. Distal chevron osteotomy with lateral release for treatment of hallux valgus deformity. Foot Ankle Int 1994; 15(9):457.
20. Schneider W, Aigner N, Pinggera O, et al. Chevron osteotomy in hallux valgus. Ten-year results of 112 cases. J Bone Joint Surg Br 2004;86(7):1016.
21. Trnka HJ, Zembsch A, Easley ME, et al. The chevron osteotomy for correction of hallux valgus. Comparison of findings after two and five years of follow-up. J Bone Joint Surg Am 2000;82(10):1373.
22. Nyska M. Principles of first metatarsal osteotomies. Foot Ankle Clin 2001;6(3):399.
23. Easley ME, Trnka HJ. Current concepts review: hallux valgus part II: operative treatment. Foot Ankle Int 2007;28(6):748.
24. Kramer J. DieKramer osteotomie zur behandlung des hallux valgus und des digitus quintus varus. Operat Orthop Traumat 2004;2:29.
25. Bosch P, Wanke S, Legenstein R. Hallux valgus correction by the method of Bosch: a new technique with a seven-to-ten-year follow-up. Foot Ankle Clin 2000;5:485.
26. Giannini S, Faldini C, Vannini F, et al. Surgical treatment of hallux valgus: a clinical prospective randomized study comparing linear distal metatarsal osteotomy with scarf osteotomy. J Bone Joint Surg Br Proceedings 2009;91.

27. Kadakia AR, Smerek JP, Myerson MS. Radiographic results after percutaneous distal metatarsal osteotomy for correction of hallux valgus deformity. Foot Ankle Int 2007;28(3):355.
28. Murawski DE, Beskin JL. Increased displacement maximizes the utility of the distal chevron osteotomy for hallux valgus deformity correction. Foot Ankle Int 2008;29(2):155.
29. Barker A. An operation of hallux valgus. Lancet 1884;1:655.
30. Lamprecht E, Kramer J. Die metatarsale-i-osteotomie nach Kramer zur behandlung des hallux valgus. Orthopraxis 1982;28:636.
31. Trnka HJ, Hofmann S, Wiesauer H, et al. Kramer versus Austin Osteotomy: two distal metatarsal osteotomies for correction of hallux valgus deformities. Orthopaed Int Ed 1997;5:110.
32. Maffulli N, Longo UG, Marinozzi A, et al. Hallux valgus: effectiveness and safety of minimally invasive surgery. A systematic review. Br Med Bull 2011;97:149.
33. Fernández de Retana P, Ortega JP, Poggio D, et al. Scarf and Akin osteotomy in comparison with SERI technique in the treatment of hallux valgus. Presented at the In: American Orthopaedic Foot and Ankle Society 23rd Annual Summer Meeting. Toronto, July 13–15, 2007.
34. Lagaay PM, Hamilton GA, Ford LA, et al. Rates of revision surgery using Chevron-Austin osteotomy, Lapidus arthrodesis, and closing base wedge osteotomy for correction of hallux valgus deformity. J Foot Ankle Surg 2008;47(4):267.
35. Viehe R, Haupt DJ, Heaslet MW, et al. Complications of screw-fixated chevron osteotomies for the correction of hallux abducto valgus. J Am Podiatr Med Assoc 2003;93(6):499.
36. Nigro JS, Greger GM, Catanzariti AR. Closing base wedge osteotomy. J Foot Surg 1991;30(5):494.
37. Gerbert J. Austin type bunionectomy. In: Gerbert J, editor. Textbook of bunion surgery. 2nd edtion. Mt Kisco (NY): Futura Publishing; 1991. p. 167–221.

Rotational and Opening Wedge Basal Osteotomies

Paulo N. Ferrao, FCS (SA) Ortho*,
Nikiforos P. Saragas, FCS (SA) Ortho, MMed (Ortho Surg)(Wits)

KEYWORDS

- Ludloff • Proximal opening wedge osteotomy • Hallux valgus • Basal osteotomies
- Rotational osteotomy

KEY POINTS

- The Ludloff and proximal opening wedge osteotomies are powerful basal rotational osteotomies, very effective in correcting moderate to severe hallux valgus deformities.
- With the advent of modern fixation options and revised surgical techniques, these osteotomies are technically easier, stable, and reproducible, representing valuable additions to the surgeon's armamentarium in approaching the complex deformity known as hallux valgus.
- Unfortunately there is no singular procedure that can address all deformities. By not stretching indications and choosing the appropriate procedure, patient satisfaction can be maximized and risks minimized.

ROTATIONAL OSTEOTOMY
Introduction

Carl Heuter[1] first described the term Hallux Valgus in 1871. Hallux valgus usually occurs from the second to fifth decade, with a peak incidence in the third decade. Coughlin and Jones[2] found that 83% of patients had a positive family history and 84% had bilateral deformities. He also found that only 34% of cases were as a result of constrictive shoes and occupation. More than 150 procedures have been described for the treatment of hallux valgus, indicating the complexity of the deformity. Treatment options are usually guided by the severity of the deformity. Moderate to severe hallux valgus has traditionally been managed with a shaft or proximal osteotomy together with distal soft-tissue release.

Proximal osteotomies can be classified as translation or rotational osteotomy, the latter of which is geometrically more powerful.[3] The commonly described proximal

Department of Orthopedic Surgery, WITS University, Jubilee Road, Johannesburg 2193, South Africa
* Corresponding author. Suite 303 Linksfield Medical Centre, 24 12th Avenue, Gauteng 2192, South Africa.
E-mail address: Paulo@cybersmart.co.za

Foot Ankle Clin N Am 19 (2014) 203–221
http://dx.doi.org/10.1016/j.fcl.2014.02.004
1083-7515/14/$ – see front matter © 2014 Elsevier Inc. All rights reserved.

foot.theclinics.com

osteotomies are the crescentic, proximal chevron, Ludloff, Mao, and opening or closing wedge. The crescentic osteotomy was popular but had its drawbacks. Technically
it is difficult to perform and to obtain stable fixation, as a result of which dorsal malunions and shortening became common, with the risk of causing transfer metatarsalgia. The literature reports up to 28% incidence of this complication.[4–8] The proximal
chevron is easy to fix but can be difficult to translate because of the proximal flare
of the first metatarsal. The Ludloff osteotomy, first described in 1918, used no fixation
for stabilization.[9] Because of the inherent instability of this osteotomy together with the
lack of fixation, it did not gain much popularity. The addition of fixation to the osteotomy by Cisar and colleagues[10] resulted in surgeons revising this procedure, and a
renewed enthusiasm followed. Trnka and colleagues[11] found the Ludloff osteotomy
to be significantly more rigid than the crescentic and proximal chevron osteotomies.
Myerson then published a modified Ludloff technique with stable fixation and good
reproducible results, which led to an increased interest in the Ludloff osteotomy and subsequent numerous publications.[12–18] The Mao osteotomy is, in essence, a reverse
Ludloff osteotomy. Although theoretically more stable, it is difficult to maintain the point
of rotation proximally enough, resulting in shortening and a bowing effect of the metatarsal. The basal opening wedge osteotomy was first described in 1923 by Trethowan,
whose technique made use of a bone block and no fixation, as he believed that maintaining the lateral cortex gave the osteotomy sufficient stability.[19] This technically demanding
procedure was abandoned due to concerns about instability and nonunions.[20,21] This
osteotomy was historically used in adolescent hallux valgus with questionable results.[22–24]
The use of a mini Hoffman external fixator, suggested by Amarnek and colleagues[25] in
the 1980s, was, as expected, not well accepted. With the advent of special opening
wedge plates, however, this procedure has started to gain favor. This article mainly
considers 2 rotational osteotomies, the Ludloff and opening wedge, although the principles are transferable to other variations of the proximal first metatarsal osteotomy.

Preoperative Assessment

All patients presenting with hallux valgus should have a thorough history and full clinical examination undertaken.

The most significant factors to be elicited from the history are:

1. Positive family history (often present).
2. Ask about the presence of any neuromuscular disorders, which is a contraindication to performing corrective osteotomies. It may be preferable to fuse the first
   metatarsophalangeal (MTP) joint.
3. Inflammatory arthropathies such as rheumatoid arthritis (RA). One must be
   cautious in these patients, as recurrence is much higher because of poor quality
   of the soft tissue. Some surgeons may argue that owing to modern-day biologics
   used in treating RA, this is no longer a relative contraindication.
4. Smoking increases the risk of nonunion in osteotomies. Myerson and colleagues
   reported that the risk of nonunion was up to 4 times higher.
5. Diabetes also increases the risk of nonunion. Shibuya and colleagues reported a
   25.4% bone-healing complication rate in diabetics undergoing foot and ankle
   surgery.[26]

The most important features of the clinical examination are:

1. Assess for the presence of arthritis in the first MTP joint. Patients with Grade 1
   (Hattrup and Johnson) hallux MTP arthritis can be managed as a hallux valgus patient. Patients with Grade 2 arthritis need to be carefully assessed, and appropriate

surgery performed according to merit. Patients with Grade 3 arthritis are better off with a fusion.

2. Confirm that the patient is symptomatic. This surgery is not cosmetic. The patient may have a pain-free abnormal-appearing hallux before surgery and end up with a beautiful-appearing hallux that is painful after surgery.
3. Assess correctability of the deformity. A very rigid deformity is suggestive of arthritis.
4. Assess for hypermobility of the first ray. These patients have a high recurrence rate with osteotomies and should rather have a modified Lapidus procedure.
5. Rule out sesamoiditis. In the mild hallux valgus deformity, painful sesamoiditis can be misdiagnosed as a painful bunion.
6. Document the neurovascular status of the foot. Be sure to document sensation to the hallux.

All patients must have full weight-bearing radiographs of the feet. Three views must be done: Anterior-posterior (AP), oblique, and lateral. Take note of the bone quality (looking specifically for osteopenia) and width of the first metatarsal. Certain osteotomies are contraindicated in the presence of a narrow metatarsal, as the osteotomy can only be translated up to a maximum of 80% of the width of the metatarsal. Thus with a narrow metatarsal the amount of correction could be inadequate. In the presence of osteopenia, supplementary fixation may be required. It is important to note the length of the first metatarsal relative to the second metatarsal. If the first metatarsal is short, one must avoid an osteotomy that will shorten it even more. The reason for this is to avoid transfer metatarsalgia.

The following angles must be measured (**Fig. 1**):

1. Hallux valgus angle (HVA)
2. 1-2 intermetatarsal angle (IMA)
3. Distal metatarsal articular angle (DMAA)
4. Sesamoid position

These angles are used to assess the severity of the deformity and classify it as mild, moderate, or severe. The most appropriate procedure can then be chosen to best correct the deformity (**Table 1**).

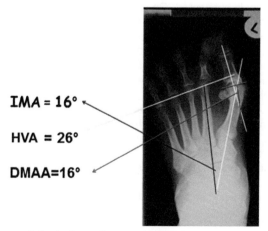

Fig. 1. Measurement of the hallux valgus angle (HVA), 1-2 intermetatarsal angle (IMA), distal metatarsal articular angle (DMAA), and sesamoid position.

Table 1
Assessment of severity of deformity

	Hallux Valgus Angle	Intermetatarsal Angle
Normal	<15°	<9°
Mild	15°–30°	9°–13°
Moderate	30°–40°	13°–20°
Severe	>40°	>20°

A detailed explanation must be given to the patient regarding what the procedure entails (illustrations are very helpful), the risks of the surgery, and the postoperative protocol.

Ludloff Osteotomy

In 1918, Ludloff[9] described an oblique osteotomy of the first metatarsal to correct metatarsus primus varus. He originally shortened the metatarsal and used no fixation. Today's modified technique is easier to perform, stable, and reproducible. This osteotomy has gained increasing popularity over the past decade.

Decision making

This osteotomy is indicated in painful hallux valgus deformities, which are by definition moderate or severe. The authors would consider the current indication to be a hallux valgus angle (HVA) greater than 35° or an intermetatarsal angle (IMA) greater than 15°.

The absolute and relative contraindications to this procedure are:

- Instability at the first metatarsocuneiform (MC) joint, assessed by manually stressing the MC joint in various directions while stabilizing the lesser toe rays. This very subjective assessment is controversial as regards its presence and diagnosis in the literature. Bednarz and Manoli[27] defined hypermobility of the first ray as more than 1 thumb-breadth of dorsal and plantar motion with the lesser toes stabilized. Myerson described taking AP radiographs of the foot with and without strapping the forefoot. If the IMA corrects with strapping of the transverse plane, instability is suspected. On weight-bearing radiographs of the feet, one should look for translation of the first metatarsal (MT) relative to the medial cuneiform on the AP view, and plantar opening of the joint on the lateral view.[16] Using these criteria, the authors recommend that if there is any suspicion of instability, a modified Lapidus procedure should be performed.
- Be cautious in patients with a narrow first metatarsal, as stable fixation can be difficult to achieve.
- A large DMAA, as this is a rotational osteotomy. The rotation will worsen the DMAA, resulting in incongruence of the joint, which can lead to arthritis or recurrence (**Fig. 2**). In these cases a translation osteotomy (eg, Scarf) or double osteotomy is preferable.
- Severe arthritis of the MTP joint. It is preferable to fuse the MTP joint in these cases.
- Trnka and colleagues[28] suggest caution in osteoporotic patients.

Surgical technique

The patient is positioned supine with a tourniquet applied to the thigh. The patient is given an ankle block using local anesthetic for postoperative pain control.

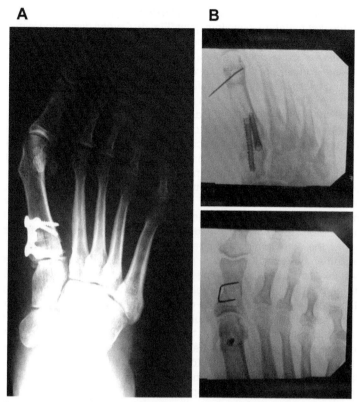

Fig. 2. (*A*) Rotational osteotomy used in the presence of an increased DMAA resulted in recurrence, which was revised with a double osteotomy (*B*). A distal medial-based wedge Chevron osteotomy was done to correct the high DMAA.

The distal lateral soft-tissue release is performed first through a dorsal incision in the first web space (**Fig. 3**). The adductor tendon is stripped off the proximal phalanx and the sesamoid suspensory ligament is transected. The capsule is then released in a pie-crust fashion until the hallux can be manipulated into 20° of varus.

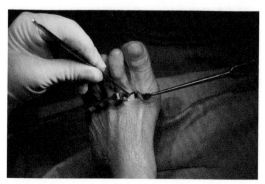

Fig. 3. The distal lateral soft-tissue release is performed first through a dorsal incision in the first web space.

Next, a longitudinal medial incision is made extending from the base of the proximal phalanx to the first metatarsocuneiform joint (**Fig. 4**). Careful dissection is made down to the capsule so as not to injure the medial dorsal cutaneous nerve. The capsule is identified by its vertically running fibers, and carefully dissected out. A capsulotomy, using an L-shaped incision, is made. A wedge of capsule is excised from the vertical limb according to the severity of the deformity and prominence of the bunion, usually about 3 to 5 mm (**Fig. 5**). It is important not to have to rely on the capsulorrhaphy for correction of the deformity. The medial bony eminence is resected parallel to the metatarsal shaft, starting just medial to the sagittal sulcus. One should be careful not to cut lateral to the sulcus, as this could cause a varus deformity to develop.

The first MC joint is identified and a mark made, using diathermy, 5 mm distal to the joint dorsally. An oblique osteotomy is marked out from this point in a dorsal proximal to plantar distal direction. The osteotomy should exit a couple of millimeters proximal to the sesamoid and have an angle of approximately 30° relative to the metatarsal shaft. One should be aware of the plantar blood supply to the metatarsal head so as not to compromise it. If the planned osteotomy will exit too close to this crucial blood supply, the osteotomy should be redirected. The osteotomy can be marked out using diathermy. A small Hohmann retractor is placed dorsally at the tarsometa-tarsal (TMT) joint to protect the extensor hallucis longus tendon, and another is placed plantar distal to protect the blood supply to the metatarsal head.[4] Start by only per-forming the proximal two-thirds of the osteotomy, as described by Myerson, using an oscillating saw. The saw blade should be aimed about 10° plantarward, so as to prevent elevation during rotation of the osteotomy.[16] This maneuver was first described by Nyska and colleagues.[3] Beischer and colleagues,[29] using 3-dimensional computer analysis of the Ludloff osteotomy, established these osteotomy guidelines as optimal.[16] The osteotomy is then loosely fixed using a 3.0- to 3.5-mm lag screw, as proximal as possible, while not compromising the fixation. The entry point for the screw is approximately 10 mm distal to the starting point of the osteotomy. Placing the screw as proximal as possible allows for correction to occur at the base of the deformity, making it more powerful and minimizing shortening.[3] The screw can be solid or cannulated headless, but must run perpendicular to the cut. It is advisable to countersink the screw head, as most case series report prominent hardware as a complication. The screw must then be backed out a few millimeters to allow the saw blade to be reintroduced. The benefit of fixing the incomplete osteotomy first is to have better control when rotating the completed osteotomy. The osteotomy is thus completed, and the distal fragment rotated laterally around the proximal fixation.

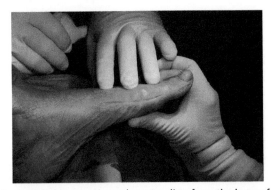

Fig. 4. A longitudinal medial incision is made, extending from the base of the proximal pha-lanx to the first metatarsocuneiform joint.

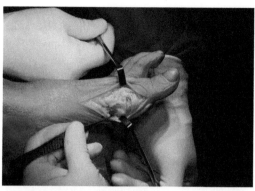

Fig. 5. A wedge of capsule is excised from the vertical limb according to the severity of the deformity and prominence of the bunion, usually about 3 to 5 mm.

The proximal fragment can be held with a towel clip to aid rotation of the distal fragment.[28] The proximal screw is tightened and reduction of the IMA confirmed under fluoroscopy. The use of imaging with this procedure is important, as it is easy to overcorrect or undercorrect the IMA. The IMA should not be reduced to less than 5°.[30] Reducing the IMA to less than 5° has the risk of causing hallux varus. Once adequate correction is achieved, a second screw is then inserted more distally across the osteotomy from plantar to dorsal. If there is space, a third screw can be inserted. The formed medial bony shelf is excised using an oscillating saw, with care being taken not to compromise the fixation.

The joint is washed out and a capsulorrhaphy performed (**Fig. 6**). The hallux is held in a neutral position and any pronation corrected while repairing the capsule. In the presence of hallux interphalangeus, an increased DMAA, or severe pronation, an Akin osteotomy can be added (**Fig. 7**). A dressing is applied and the foot bandaged so as to hold the hallux in a neutral position.

Postoperative protocol
The patient can be mobilized in a postoperative heel-bearing wedge shoe so as not to stress the osteotomy. The patient is instructed to have strict elevation of the operated leg and minimal mobilization during the first 2 weeks, to minimize swelling and allow for wound healing. Thereafter the patient can be more mobile in the wedge shoe. The dressing is changed at weeks 1, 2, 4, and 6. At each dressing change the position of the hallux is assessed and adjusted accordingly, using tape. At 6 weeks radiographs are taken to assess alignment and bony union. The Ludloff osteotomy should heal with primary bone healing. If callus formation is seen, this is suggestive of motion and loss of stability, which can result in shortening and dorsal malunion. These patients require prolonged immobilization in the wedge shoe to protect the osteotomy while it heals. Because of the broad surface area of bony contact, nonunions are rare. If radiographic findings are favorable, the patient is allowed to transition into comfortable supportive shoes. Impact activities are restricted for a further 4 weeks.

BASAL OPENING WEDGE OSTEOTOMY
Decision Making

This procedure is indicated in symptomatic moderate to severe hallux valgus deformities, with an HVA greater than 30° and an IMA greater than 13°. Contraindications are similar to those for the Ludloff, with exception of the increased DMAA.

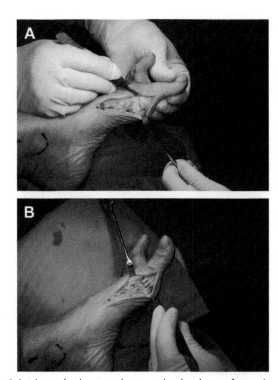

Fig. 6. (*A, B*) The joint is washed out and a capsulorrhaphy performed.

Although this is a viable method of severe hallux valgus correction, the authors have some concerns about this procedure that should be borne in mind on considering its use. It can be difficult to maintain correction and achieve stability of fixation if the lateral cortex is violated. As opposed to other translational and rotational methods of hallux valgus correction, nonunion is a more likely complication, as it is an opening wedge osteotomy. The authors believe that bone grafting is essential to achieving optimum reproducible results. An opening wedge osteotomy increases the length of the first metatarsal, which may cause increased pressure in the first MTP joint. It is not

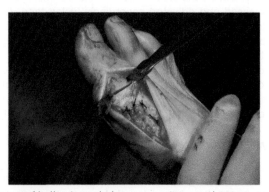

Fig. 7. In the presence of hallux interphalangeus, an increased DMAA, or severe pronation, an Akin osteotomy can be added.

known whether there are any long-term effects to the joint resulting from this procedure, to date no long-term consequences have been reported in the literature.

Surgical Technique

The patient is positioned supine with a tourniquet applied to the thigh. Some investigators suggest not using a tourniquet to minimize postoperative swelling. An ankle block is performed for postoperative pain control.

First, the distal soft-tissue release is performed through a dorsal incision in the first web space, as described earlier. A medial midline incision is made extending from the midpoint of the proximal phalanx proximally along the shaft of the first metatarsal to the first MC joint. Soft tissues should be carefully dissected off the medial capsule to protect all neurovascular structures. Periosteal stripping of the metatarsal should be minimized so as not to compromise bone healing. Once again an L-shaped capsulotomy is performed. Two parallel vertical incisions are made, 2 mm proximal to the metatarsal articular surface, which will form the wedge of capsule that is excised. On should always err on taking less and resecting more if needed when doing the capsulorrhaphy. The dorsal horizontal limb is then cut and the joint exposed (**Fig. 8**).

The bunion is excised using an oscillating saw, starting just medial to the sulcus and running parallel to the shaft. The first MC joint is identified using a 22-gauge needle. A mark is placed 1 cm distal to the joint on the metatarsal (**Fig. 9**). A transverse osteotomy is performed at this level, with extreme care taken not to violate the lateral cortex; this is technically the most difficult part of the procedure and not always possible. The intact lateral cortex acts as a hinge around which the osteotomy rotates, thereby providing inherent stability to the osteotomy. Some investigators prefer an oblique osteotomy directed at the base, believing that the dense soft-tissue attachment at the base will add stability to the lateral hinge.[31] The osteotomy is then carefully opened using 1 or 2 osteotomes (**Fig. 10**). Some sets have special devices to open the osteotomy. The size of wedge needed to correct the deformity is checked under fluoroscopy. There are reference tables offering guidance on the size of wedge needed to correct the deformity according to the IMA. Ultimately, correction must be confirmed under fluoroscopic control. The use of fluoroscopy during the procedure is once again of utmost importance. The appropriate wedge plate is applied and secured (**Fig. 11**). The worry with this osteotomy has always been the risk of nonunion, being an opening wedge osteotomy. The authors advocate inserting bone graft into the osteotomy site (**Fig. 12**). The resected medial eminence is a readily available source of bone graft.

Because of uncertainty arising from the effect on the MTP joint caused by lengthening the metatarsal, Siekmann suggested a distal shortening chevron osteotomy

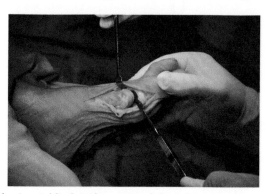

Fig. 8. The dorsal horizontal limb is then cut and the joint exposed.

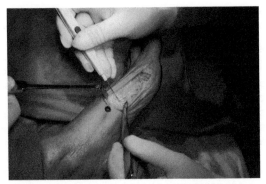

Fig. 9. A mark is placed 1 cm distal to the joint on the metatarsal.

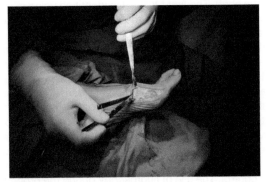

Fig. 10. The osteotomy is then carefully opened using 1 or 2 osteotomes.

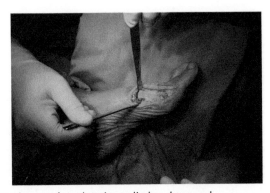

Fig. 11. The appropriate wedge plate is applied and secured.

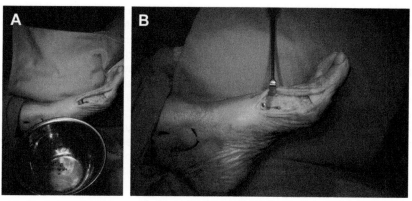

Fig. 12. (A, B) Inserting bone graft into the osteotomy site.

(the so-called double osteotomy). A normal chevron is performed with the addition of removing a 2-mm wedge block from the dorsal cut (**Fig. 13**), thus negating the lengthening effect of the osteotomy. The chevron is secured using a headless compression screw. In experienced hands this extra osteotomy should not add more than about

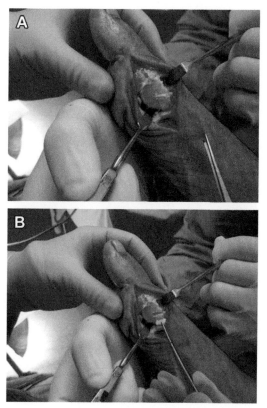

Fig. 13. (A, B) A normal chevron is performed with the addition of removing a 2-mm wedge block from the dorsal cut.

10 minutes to the surgery time. There are some added benefits from doing this second osteotomy. The resected bone is an excellent bone graft for the proximal osteotomy site. A high DMAA is usually a contraindication to rotational osteotomies. By taking a medially based wedge from the chevron an increased DMAA can be corrected (**Fig. 14**), thus increasing the indications for this osteotomy.

The joint is then washed out. The capsule is repaired using Vicryl while holding the hallux in a neutral position and rotation. If there is residual interphalangeus or severe pronation of the hallux, an Akin osteotomy is performed. The wound is closed with subcuticular absorbable sutures (Quill; Angiotech, Vancouver, BC, Canada). The authors believe that using subcuticular sutures causes fewer wound-healing problems and saves time at follow-up, as sutures do not have to be removed. The foot is bandaged so as to maintain the hallux in a neutral position (**Fig. 15**).

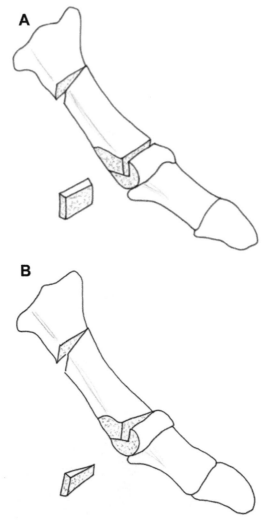

Fig. 14. (*A, B*) By taking a medially based wedge from the chevron, an increased DMAA can be corrected.

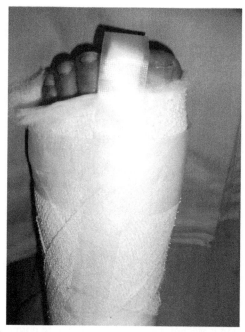

Fig. 15. The foot is bandaged so as to maintain the hallux in a neutral position.

Postoperative Protocol

The patient can be mobilized in a postoperative heel-bearing wedge shoe so as not to stress the osteotomy. The follow-up protocol is similar to that with a Ludloff osteotomy. At 6 weeks radiographs are taken to assess alignment, correction, and bony union with incorporation of the bone graft. Callus formation seen along the lateral cortex indicates disruption of the lateral cortex, which can decrease stability of the fixation with mobility at the osteotomy site. These patients are protected for a further 2 weeks in the wedge shoe and followed up closely for delayed union. Once bony union is evident, patients can transition to normal shoes (**Fig. 16**).

DISCUSSION

The true etiology behind the hallux valgus deformity is still poorly understood and heatedly debated. As a result, more than a 150 procedures have been described in attempting to address the deformity. All proximal osteotomies are at risk of developing recurrence, hallux varus, joint stiffness, malunion, nonunion, and infection.[32] The surgeon has therefore to decide on which osteotomy best corrects the deformity with the least risk of complications. Mann and Coughlin popularized the basal crescentic osteotomy, with good results in even severe deformities.[21,33] The drawback with proximal osteotomies such as the crescentic, besides being technically difficult, is dorsal malunions and transfer metatarsalgia, which has been documented in many studies.[13,33–37] Some investigators believe that dorsal malunions occur more commonly in proximal osteotomies done through a dorsal incision, such as the crescentic and closing wedge osteotomies.[6,16,36] Dorsal angulation has been reported to be as high as 82% in the literature.[35] The recent literature reports a very low incidence

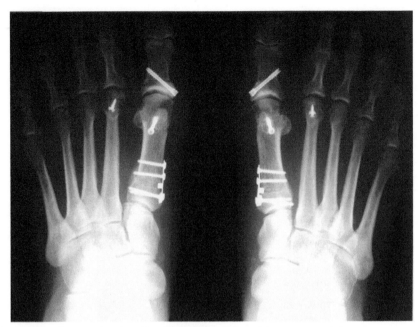

Fig. 16. Once bony union is evident, patients can transition to normal shoes.

of this complication with the Ludloff osteotomy, which allows for a broad area of bony metaphyseal contact giving better stability and healing.

Chiodo and colleagues[16] reviewed 70 cases of patients who had a Ludloff osteotomy to correct moderate to severe hallux valgus. The average HVA and IMA were corrected from 31° and 16° preoperatively to 11° and 7° postoperatively. The metatarsal was plantarflexed 1° on average and shortened by 2.3 mm. Complications consisted of prominent hardware in 5, hallux varus in 4, delayed unions in 3, and superficial infections in 4 patients. There were no patients with transfer metatarsalgia, a finding in contrast to those of similar studies evaluating the crescentic osteotomy.[37–39] This result is most likely because the osteotomy actually plantarflexed the first metatarsal. Chiodo's group found an association between delayed union and steepness of the osteotomy. There was a 98% satisfaction rate.[16]

Trnka and colleagues[28] reported on 111 Ludloff procedures having 80% good to excellent results. There was significant improvement in the American Orthopaedic Foot and Ankle Society (AOFAS) scores. Of note, patients younger than 60 years were happier with the procedure than patients older than 60. The IMA was corrected from 17° to 8°. Complications included 4 recurrences (2 of which showed radiologic features of TMT instability) and 9 hallux varus (only 2 were symptomatic); 5 patients had prominent hardware and a 2% incidence of delayed union. The authors suspect that the shorter the osteotomy, the less stable the fixation becomes. There was no incidence of dorsal malunion, and a mean shortening of 2.2 mm.[16] Saxena and McCammon[40] reported only 1.4 mm of shortening and no dorsal malunion in their earlier series.

Chiodo and colleagues[16] and Trnka and colleagues[28] reported 7% and 3% incidence of prominent hardware, respectively, significantly less than the incidence with crescentic osteotomies, which is reported to be as high as 52%.[6,16,37,38] By using headless compression screws this complication can be markedly reduced. Some surgeons prefer using a standard cortical screw for proximal fixation. In these instances the head should be countersunk to minimize prominence of the hardware.

Saxena and McCammon[40] reported on the use of a medial locking plate in a comparison with screw fixation, with similar results in correction and satisfaction. These plates could be of use in patients with osteoporotic bone or a narrow first metatarsal. Both of these instances are reported to be at risk for developing instability with screw fixation. In the event of an intraoperative fracture whereby screw fixation is no longer possible, a locking plate is very useful. Additional fixation is described in the literature to improve stability and allow for earlier mobilization. Stamatis and colleagues[41] described the addition of a mini locking plate as a buttress in addition to the screws, although they do not mention the incidence of prominent hardware, which could be higher with this technique. Schon and colleagues[42] described the use of 1 or 2 Kirschner wires from the proximal medial surface down the shaft of the distal segment in cases where the second screw fixation is not adequate. Stamatis and colleagues[43] demonstrated adequate fixation using threaded Kirschner wires in a biomechanical cadaver study.

Hofstaetter and colleagues[19] showed in a cadaver study that there was no difference in fixation strength when comparing normal cortical screws with headless screws, and also showed that the Ludloff osteotomy fixed with 2 screws is mechanically superior to the opening wedge plate with regard to weight bearing. Fixation of the proximal opening wedge osteotomy has also been of concern in the past. With the advent of specialized low-profile plates, this is no longer an issue. Shurnas and colleagues[31,44] showed that the proximal opening wedge osteotomy fixed with a plate is as stable as the proximal chevron osteotomy. Hofstaetter and colleagues,[19] in their cadaver study, stated that lateral cortex integrity and good bone density were important factors in achieving a satisfactorily stable fixation of the proximal opening wedge osteotomy.

Shurnas and colleagues[31] reported on 84 proximal opening wedge osteotomies. The HVA improved from 30° preoperatively to 10° postoperatively on average. There was an average of 3° correction per 1 mm of opening the osteotomy. The IMA improved from 14.5° preoperatively to 4.6° postoperatively on average. The visual analog scale improved from 5.9 to 0.5. Complications consisted of 1 nonunion, 1 delayed union, 4 hallux varus, and 3 recurrences. Disruption of the lateral cortex (12% of cases) had no adverse consequences, such as loss of correction, fixation failure, or first-ray elevation or shortening. These findings are contrary to those in other literature.[45–47] Lengthening of the first ray averaged 1.9 mm, which was not statistically significant. Range of motion was not affected, disproving theories that the lengthening would cause "jamming" of the joint and eventual arthritis. Moreover, a biplanar distal chevron osteotomy was suggested for cases with an increased DMAA.[44]

Saragas[46] reported an improvement in the AOFAS forefoot score from 51.3 to 86.8 in 64 moderate hallux valgus deformities that had a proximal opening wedge osteotomy. There was a mean increase in the first metatarsal length of 2.3 mm, which was also not statistically significant. Complications consisted of 5 hallux varus (1 symptomatic), 2 asymptomatic recurrences, 2 cases of prominent hardware, and 1 nonunion.

Randhawa and Pepper[39] reported on 25 proximal opening wedge osteotomies. This series showed improvements in the HVA from 45.5° to 13.1° and in the IMA from 17.7° to 9.2°. There was an 80% satisfaction rate. Complications consisted of 1 hallux varus, 1 nonunion (asymptomatic), and 1 recurrence. Wukich and colleagues[48] reviewed 18 cases and reported an 89% satisfaction rate. The HVA improved by 13.5° and the IMA by 9°, post correction on average. The 23 patients in the series of Cooper and colleagues[45] achieved a mean correction of 15° for the HVA and 7° for the IMA. There were 2 recurrences, 1 wound problem, and 1 delayed union.

Hallux varus is the most common complication in most studies, resulting from overcorrection; this indicates the inbuilt power of correction of the proximal opening wedge osteotomy. It is prudent to use intraoperative fluoroscopy during surgery before deciding on the final wedge size. The other concern with proximal opening wedge osteotomy is that it lengthens the first metatarsal. Budny and colleagues[49] performed an in vitro study to assess the amount of lengthening that is geometrically inherent to proximal opening wedge osteotomy. He reported a 1% to 2.8% increase in total length attributable to the osteotomy. Of interest was that there was no difference in lengthening whether the osteotomy was transverse or oblique. Whether this lengthening is of any clinical significance is the concern.[46,50] Some investigators believe that the lengthening created with opening wedge osteotomy results in tightening of the soft tissue, which can result in a higher rate of recurrence.[31,45] Others consider that it can cause so-called "jamming" of the MTP joint that would eventually result in arthritis. It would require long-term follow-up to confirm or disprove these theories. The addition of the distal shortening chevron osteotomy has negated these concerns about lengthening the first metatarsal, with added benefits. The use of the resected bone wedge as bone graft makes it unnecessary to harvest bone, which might have put surgeons off using this osteotomy. In revision cases where previous surgery has resulted in shortening of the first metatarsal, the lengthening effect of the proximal opening wedge osteotomy is advantageous. This minimal lengthening also prevents the risk of transfer metatarsalgia. By taking a medially based wedge from the chevron osteotomy an increased DMAA can be corrected, thus broadening the indications for use of the proximal opening wedge osteotomy.

When performing a proximal opening wedge osteotomy, most investigators emphasize maintaining the lateral cortex for stability. Breaking the lateral cortex could result in instability of the conventional fixation, thus increasing the risk of nonunion and even leading to loss of correction. The use of new locking plates in these instances may overcome this problem.

SUMMARY

The Ludloff and proximal opening wedge osteotomies are powerful basal rotational osteotomies that are very effective in correcting moderate to severe hallux valgus deformities. With the advent of modern fixation options and revised surgical techniques, these osteotomies are technically easier, stable, and reproducible, representing valuable additions to the surgeon's armamentarium in approaching the complex deformity known as hallux valgus. Unfortunately there is no perfect procedure that can address all deformities. By not stretching indications and choosing the appropriate procedure, patient satisfaction can be maximized and risks minimized.

REFERENCES

1. Donley BG, Vaughn RA, Stephenson KA, et al. Keller resection arthroplasty for treatment of hallux valgus deformity: increased correction with fibular sesamoidectomy. Foot Ankle Int 2002;23:699–703.
2. Coughlin MJ, Jones CP. Demographics, etiology, and radiographic assessment. Foot Ankle Int 2007;28:759–77.
3. Nyska M, Trnka HJ, Parks BG, et al. Proximal metatarsal osteotomies: a comparative geometric analysis conducted on sawbone models. Foot Ankle Int 2002;23: 938–45.

4. Trnka HJ, Hofstaetter SG, Hofstaetter JG, et al. Intermediate-term results of the Ludloff osteotomy in one hundred and eleven feet. J Bone Joint Surg Am 2008; 90:531–9.
5. Mann RA. Distal soft tissue procedure and proximal metatarsal osteotomy for correction of hallux valgus deformity. Orthopedics 1990;13:1013–8.
6. Easley ME, Kiebzak GM, Davis WH, et al. Prospective, randomized comparison of proximal crescentic and proximal chevron osteotomies for correction of hallux valgus deformity. Foot Ankle Int 1996;17:307–16.
7. Brodsky JW, Beischer A, Robinson A, et al. Hallux valgus correction with modified McBride bunionectomy and proximal crescentic osteotomy: clinical, radiologic and pedobarographic outcome. Presented at the 31st Annual Meeting of the American Orthopaedic Foot and Ankle Society. San Francisco, March 3, 2001.
8. Zettl R, Trnka HJ, Easley M, et al. Moderate to severe hallux valgus deformity: correction with proximal crescentic osteotomy and distal soft tissue release. Arch Orthop Trauma Surg 2000;120:397–402.
9. Ludloff K. Die Beseitigung des Hallux Valgus durch die schraege planta-dorsale Osteotomie des Metatarsus. I. Langenbecks Arch Klin Chir Ver Dtsch Z Chir 1918;110:364–87.
10. Cisar J, Holz U, Jenninger W, et al. Die Osteotomie nach Ludloff bei der Hallux-valgus-Operation. [Ludloff's osteotomy in hallux valgus surgery]. Aktuelle Traumatol 1983;13:247–9 [in German].
11. Trnka HJ, Parks BG, Ivanic G, et al. Six first metatarsal shaft osteotomies: mechanical and immobilization comparisons. Clin Orthop 2000;381:256–65.
12. Acevedo JI. Fixation of metatarsal osteotomies in the treatment of hallux valgus. Foot Ankle Clin 2000;5(3):451–68.
13. Acevedo JI, Sammarco VJ, Boucher HR, et al. Mechanical comparison of cyclic loading in five different first metatarsal shaft osteotomies. Foot Ankle Int 2002;23: 711–6.
14. Basile A, Battaglia A, Campi A. Retrospective analysis of the Ludloff osteotomy for correction of severe hallux valgus deformity. Foot Ankle Surg 2001;7:1–8.
15. Chao W, Mizel MS. Specialty update: what's new in foot and ankle surgery. J Bone Joint Surg Am 2006;88:909–22.
16. Chiodo CP, Schon LC, Myerson MS. Clinical results with the Ludloff osteotomy for correction of adult hallux valgus. Foot Ankle Int 2004;25:532–6.
17. Hofstaetter SG, Gruber F, Ritschl P, et al. The modified Ludloff osteotomy for correction of severe metatarsus primus varus with hallux valgus deformity. Z Orthop Ihre Grenzgeb 2006;144:141–7.
18. Petroutsas J, Trnka HJ. The Ludloff osteotomy for correction of hallux valgus. Oper Orthop Traumatol 2005;17:102–7.
19. Hofstaetter SG, Glisson RR, Alitz CJ, et al. Biomechanical comparison of screws and plates for hallux valgus opening-wedge and Ludloff osteotomies. Clin Biomech (Bristol, Avon) 2008;23(1):101–8. http://dx.doi.org/10.1016/j.Clinbiomech. 2007.08.012.
20. Coughlin MJ. Hallux valgus. J Bone Joint Surg Am 1996;78(6):932–66.
21. Mann RA, Coughlin MJ. Adult hallux valgus. In: Coughlin MJ, Mann RA, editors. Surgery of the foot and ankle, vol. 1, 7th edition. St Louis (MO): Mosby; 1999. p. 150–269.
22. Bonney G, Macnab I. Hallux valgus and hallux rigidus; a critical survey of operative results. J Bone Joint Surg Br 1952;34(3):366–85.
23. Scranton PE, Zuckerman JD. Bunion surgery in adolescents: results of surgical treatment. J Pediatr Orthop 1984;4(1):39–43.

24. Simmonds FA, Menelaus MB. Hallux valgus in adolescents. J Bone Joint Surg Br 1960;42(4):761–8.
25. Amarnek DL, Juda EJ, Oloff LM, et al. Opening base wedge osteotomy of the first metatarsal utilizing rigid external fixation. J Foot Surg 1986;25(4):321–6.
26. Shibuya N, Humphers JM, Fluhman BL, et al. Factors associated with nonunion, delayed union, and malunion in foot and ankle surgery in diabetic patients. J Foot Ankle Surg 2013;52(2):207–11.
27. Bednarz PA, Manoli A. Modified lapidus procedure for the treatment of hypermobile hallux valgus. Foot Ankle 2000;21(10):816–21.
28. Trnka HJ, Hofstaetter SG, Easley ME. Intermediate-term results of the Ludloff osteotomy in one hundred and eleven feet. J Bone Joint Surg Am 2009;91(Suppl 2 (Part 1)):156–68.
29. Beischer AD, Ammon P, Corniou A, et al. Three-dimensional computer analysis of the modified Ludloff osteotomy. Foot Ankle Int 2005;26(8):627–32.
30. Bae SY, Schon LC. Surgical strategies: Ludloff first metatarsal osteotomy. Foot Ankle Int 2007;28:137–44.
31. Shurnas PS, Watson TS, Crislip TW. Proximal first metatarsal opening wedge osteotomy with a low profile plate. Foot Ankle Int 2009;30:865–72.
32. Easley ME, Trnka HJ. Current concepts review: hallux valgus part II: operative treatment. Foot Ankle Int 2007;28:748–58.
33. Mann RA, Rudicel S, Graves SC. Repair of hallux valgus with a distal soft-tissue procedure and proximal metatarsal osteotomy; a long term follow-up. J Bone Joint Surg Am 1992;74-A:124–9.
34. Neese OJ, Zelichowski JE, Patton GW. Mau osteotomy: an alternative procedure to the closing abductory base wedge osteotomy. J Foot Surg 1989;28:352–62.
35. Pearson SW, Kitaoka HB, Cracchiolo A III, et al. Results and complications following a proximal curved osteotomy of the hallux metatarsal. Contemp Orthop 1991;23:127–32.
36. Sammarco GJ, Brainard BJ, Sammarco VJ. Bunion correction using proximal Chevron osteotomy. Foot Ankle 1993;14:8–14.
37. Thordarson DB, Leventen EO. Hallux valgus correction with proximal metatarsal osteotomy: two-year follow-up. Foot Ankle 1992;13:321–6.
38. Markbreiter LA, Thompson FM. Proximal metatarsal osteotomy in hallux valgus correction: a comparison of crescentic and chevron procedures. Foot Ankle Int 1997;18:71–6.
39. Randhawa S, Pepper D. Radiographic evaluation of hallux valgus treated with opening wedge osteotomy. Foot Ankle Int 2009;30:427–31.
40. Saxena A, McCammon D. The Ludloff osteotomy: a critical analysis. J Foot Ankle Surg 1997;36:100–5, 159–60.
41. Stamatis ED, Chatzikomninos LE, Karaoglanis GC. Mini locking plate as 'medial buttress' for oblique osteotomy for hallux valgus. Foot Ankle Int 2010;31:920–2.
42. Schon LC, Dom KJ, Jung HG. Clinical tip: stabilization of the proximal Ludloff osteotomy. Foot Ankle Int 2005;26:579.
43. Stamatis ED, Navid DO, Parks BG, et al. Strength of fixation of Ludloff metatarsal osteotomy utilizing three different types of Kirschner wires: a biomechanical study. Foot Ankle Int 2003;24(10):805–11.
44. Shurnas PS. Proximal opening wedge osteotomy of the first metatarsal: biomechanical and clinical evaluation. Proceedings of the AAOS annual meeting, specialty day. Chicago: 2006.
45. Cooper MT, Berlet GC, Shurnas PS, et al. Proximal opening-wedge osteotomy of the first metatarsal for correction of hallux valgus. Surg Technol Int 2007;16:215–9.

46. Saragas NP. Proximal opening-wedge osteotomy of the first metatarsal for hallux valgus using a low profile plate. Foot Ankle Int 2009;30:976–80.
47. Kumar S, Konan S, Oddy MJ, et al. Basal medial opening wedge first metatarsal osteotomy stabilized with a low profile wedge plate. Acta Orthop Belg 2012;78(3): 362–8.
48. Wukich DK, Roussel AJ, Dial DM. Correction of metatarsus primus varus with an opening wedge plate: a review of 18 procedures. J Foot Ankle Surg 2009 Jul-Aug;48(4):420–6.
49. Budny AM, Masadeh SB, Lyons MC 2nd, et al. The opening base wedge osteotomy and subsequent lengthening of the first metatarsal: an in vitro study. J Foot Ankle Surg 2009 Nov-Dec;48(6):662–7.
50. Limbird TJ, Da Silva RM, Groen NE. Osteotomy of the first metatarsal base for metatarsus primus varus. Foot Ankle 1989;9(4):158–62.

The Modified Lapidus Fusion

Timo Schmid, MD, Fabian Krause, MD*

KEYWORDS

- Hallux valgus • Modified Lapidus procedure • Metatarsocuneiform fusion
- Technique

KEY POINTS

- Due to its very proximal correction site and long lever arm, the Lapidus fusion, modified or not, is a powerful technique to correct hallux valgus deformities.
- The disadvantages are a high complication rate and a long postoperative rehabilitation period. Therefore, it is currently only performed in 5% to 10% of all hallux valgus deformity corrections.
- Lapidus fusion remains an important procedure, especially in moderate to severe deformities with intermetatarsal angles more than 14°, hypermobility of the first ray, arthritis of the first tarsometatarsal joint (TMTJ), and recurrent deformities.
- Every surgeon dealing with forefoot deformities encounters cases when the Lapidus procedure is a viable option.

INTRODUCTION: NATURE OF THE PROBLEM

In 1911 and more than 20 years before Lapidus published his technique, Albrecht[1] first described a first metatarsocuneiform fusion for correction of hallux valgus deformity. In 1925, Truslow[2] introduced the term, *metatarsus primus varus*, pointing out that the primary deformity of the hallux valgus in these cases is located at the proximal end of the first ray. He stated that any operative procedure that does not incorporate the correction of the deformity at its proximal origin is unscientific and inadequate. In 1932, Kleinberg[3] identified the obliquity of the first TMTJ and the consequent adduction of the first metatarsal as the ultimate cause in the etiology of hallux valgus.

It was not until 1934 that Lapidus described his technique. And although Lapidus himself stressed that he did not introduce a new principle, it is his name that is closely connected to the procedure.[4]

The original technique consisted of an arthrodesis of the first cuneiform-metatarsal joint and the first intermetatarsal joint. The fixation was achieved by simply sewing the

Department of Orthopaedic Surgery, Inselspital, University of Berne, Freiburgstrasse, Bern 3010, Switzerland
* Corresponding author.
E-mail address: fabian.krause@insel.ch

Foot Ankle Clin N Am 19 (2014) 223–233
http://dx.doi.org/10.1016/j.fcl.2014.02.005
1083-7515/14/$ – see front matter © 2014 Elsevier Inc. All rights reserved.

joint capsules with catgut. Later, fixation by crossed screws was introduced by Clark and colleagues[5] and led to a modified technique without intermetatarsal fusion.

Despite Truslow's statement, the original or the modified Lapidus technique is done in barely 10% of all hallux valgus corrections. This is likely due to a longer postoperative rehabilitation period and a higher complication rate as opposed to other techniques, particularly more distal procedures. The Lapidus procedure is a technically demanding operation: with its long lever arm, the procedure is prone to over- or undercorrection and nonunion.[6]

INDICATIONS/CONTRAINDICATIONS

According to most investigators, a distal bunion procedure is thought insufficient when the intermetatarsal angle exceeds 15° (**Table 1**). Any type of proximal metatarsal osteotomy or the more proximal tarsometatarsal arthrodesis is preferred in these cases.

Hypermobility of the first ray in the TMTJ, as originally suggested by Morton in 1928,[7] continues to be an important indication. Proper measurement of this instability remains, however, difficult. Plantar gapping of the first TMTJ on a lateral weightbearing radiograph seems to be a reliable sign. Clinical evaluation is highly subjective, however, and objective measurement with external calipers is inconvenient in daily practice.[8,9]

Hallux valgus deformity with accompanying arthritis of the first TMTJ can be treated by one single procedure with a Lapidus fusion.

Recurrence after hallux valgus correction is a difficult situation for both patient and surgeon. The Lapidus procedure can provide good correction and high satisfaction rates in this setting.[10,11]

Because the epiphysis of the basis of the first metatarsal contributes to approximately 50% of the length growth of the first ray,[12] a juvenile hallux with open epiphysis is a contraindication.

Potential athletic activity has to be taken into consideration, because only 30% of athletes with a stiffened first ray return to their preoperative level of activity after a metatarsocuneiform fusion. In contrast, 75% of the more sedentary patients achieve this goal.[13] Arthritis of the adjacent joints (eg, first metatarsophalangeal joint [MTPJ]

Table 1 Indications/contraindications		
	Indications	**Comments**
Frequent	Moderate to severe deformity Hypermobility of the first ray Generalized hyperlaxity	Intermetatarsal angle >15° Plantar gapping of TMTJ 1 on lateral radiograph Beighton score >5
Rare	Recurrent hallux valgus Juvenile hallux valgus TMT 1 arthritis	Satisfaction rate 80% Only when growth plate is closed
	Contraindications	**Comments**
Absolute	Arthritis of the first MTPJ Juvenile hallux valgus	Open growth plate
Relative	Short first metatarsal Young active patient Smoker	Consider bone block interposition Only 30% achieve preoperative activity level Higher nonunion rate

and naviculocuneiform) is a relative contraindication because the restricted motion and the enlarged lever arm may lead to an aggravation of a preexisting arthritis.

The Lapidus procedure should be used cautiously in smokers because smoking has proved to negatively influence the union rate.

Even with accurate joint denudement, there is shortening of the first ray. Therefore, a preexistent short first metatarsal is a relative contraindication. With a bone block interposition, a surgeon can overcome this shortening.[6,14]

SURGICAL TECHNIQUE/PROCEDURE
Preoperative Planning

Prior to the Lapidus procedure, a complete and thorough history, clinical examination, and radiographic work-up are mandatory. The following points are useful to determine whether a Lapidus procedure is a good option:

- Pain at the medial Lisfranc joint indicating Lisfranc arthritis, general hyperlaxity, an older sedentary patient, and recurrence after previous hallux valgus correction support a Lapidus procedure.
- Pain in the first MTPJ indicating first MTPJ arthritis, an athletic activity, and nicotine abuse should lead to consideration of other options.
- Clinical examination aims to detect a first ray hypermobility or a generalized hypermobility. Morton first described how to test the first TMTJ instability: with the patient sitting, the knee flexed and the ankle in neutral position, one hand stabilizes the lateral 4 metatarsals, whereas the other hand moves the first ray from dorsomedial to plantar-lateral. The mobility is compared with the contralateral side.[7] This subjective method, however, was shown invalid.[15] To more objectively quantify hypermobility, external calipers, like the Klaue device, may be used.[16] With this device, the first metatarsal head was elevated 9.3 mm (±1.9 mm) in patients with a hallux valgus as opposed to 5.4 (±1.4 mm) in the control group in a clinical study.

Intractable plantar keratoses underneath the second metatarsal head or on the dorsum of the first metatarsal head also indicate first TMTJ instability. The measurement of this instability, however, remains imprecise and subjective.

- General joint laxity can be estimated with a Beighton score, which consists of 9 stability assessments: ability to put the hands flat on the ground with straight knees (1 point), hyperextending both elbows (each 1 point) and knees (each 1 point), and bending both thumbs back on the front of the forearms (each 1 point) and both little fingers 90° to the back of the hands (each 1 point).[17] A score of 5 or more indicates significant ligamentous instability.
- Tenderness under palpation and passive motion indicates arthritis of the first TMTJ and the first MTPJ.
- Radiographic work-up consists of weight-bearing dorsoplantar and lateral radiographs. A severe deformity with an intermetatarsal angle greater than 15° and arthritis of the first TMTJ on the dorsoplantar view supports a Lapidus procedure. In contrast, a short first metatarsal, an open growth plate, and arthritis of the first MTP joint are contraindications. Regarding first ray hypermobility, Morton[7] stated that bony hypertrophy of the second metatarsal indicates instability of the first TMTJ, but Grebing and Coughlin[18] were not able to confirm this finding. No association of second metatarsal shaft width and medial cortical hypertrophy with hallux valgus, first ray mobility, or first metatarsal length was seen.

Normally, the first metatarsocuneiform joint is orientated slightly medial, but occasionally it may have an excessive degree of medial inclination. This leads to a metatarsus primus varus deformity, and a hallux valgus deformity is more common.[2,19–22]

In approximately 8% of patients, an os intermetatarseum is present.[8] It is often accompanied by a rigid first tarsometatarsal articulation that blocks reduction of the 1 to 2 intermetatarsal angle by distal soft tissue repair or distal metatarsal osteotomy and may indicate a Lapidus procedure.

- In approximately 20% of cases of moderate to severe hallux valgus deformity, a gap of the plantar aspect of the first TMTJ on the lateral view is seen that is associated with hallux valgus or first metatarsocuneiform joint instability.[8,9,23] It is obvious in a majority of cases and an objective sign for the often-quoted first ray instability.

Authors' Preferred Technique

The patient is placed in a supine position, sometimes with a bolster under the ipsilateral buttock allowing correct rotation of the foot. Appropriate visualization and safe dissection are ensured either by a sterile Esmarch rubber bandage at the ankle level or a tourniquet inflated to 350 mm Hg at the thigh.

- The first TMTJ is approached through a 5-cm longitudinal incision centered over the dorsomedial aspect of the joint. The accompanying distal soft tissue procedure is performed via a 3- to 4-cm longitudinal incision centered between the first and second MTPJs and a 3- to 4-cm longitudinal incision on the medial aspect of the first MTPJ.

A release of the adductor tendon and the transverse metatarsal ligament is carried out in the first web space. The lateral MTPJ capsule is perforated with several puncture wounds and disrupted by medial angulation of the toe. Medially, the joint capsule is prepared and opened horizontally and the medial bony eminence is removed. The removal of the eminence is a standard step with a resection of 2 to 4 mm in width, superior more than inferior, and without violating the medial sesamoid groove.

The joint capsule of the first TMTJ is approached retracting the extensor hallucis longus tendon laterally. The joint is opened dorsally and medially. If a fusion of the bases of the first and second metatarsal is planned, the joint is approached via the interval between the extensor halluces longus and brevis tendons. Care has to be taken not to harm the neurovascular bundle (the dorsalis pedis artery and deep peroneal nerve).

- The joint is exposed with 2 Hohmann retractors to protect the anterior tibial tendon on the medial side and the neurovascular bundle on the lateral side. With an osteotome and a small curette, the articular cartilage is completely removed. The joint is sinusoidal-shaped and 30 mm in height. Therefore, removing all cartilage of the plantar lateral aspect can be somewhat difficult. A small lamina spreader or a Kirschner wire distractor is useful to better expose the most plantar part of the joint. By resection of a small plantarly and laterally based wedge, better correction of excessive valgus and mild plantar flexion is achieved (**Fig. 1**). Alternatively, a minimal saw cut at the articular surface of the cuneiform with a small plantarly and laterally based wedge can be done if the first metatarsal is not already short.
- For a fusion of the first intermetatarsal joint, the corresponding articular surfaces are also prepared (as discussed previously). During this dissection, the penetrating branch of the dorsalis pedis artery has to be protected. Usually the authors prefer the modified Lapidus technique with simple fusion of the first

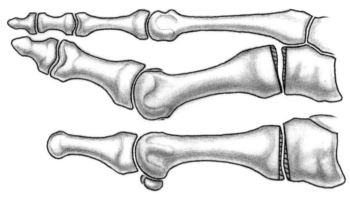

Fig. 1. By resection of a small plantarly and laterally based wedge, better correction of excessive valgus and mild plantar flexion is achieved.

TMTJ and only perform this intermetatarsal arthrodesis in cases of a nonunion or presence of an os intermetatarseum.

- The subchondral bone is opened by feathering with an osteotome and multiple 1.5-mm drill holes on both sides of the arthrodesis.
- The joint is gently manipulated from a dorsomedial to a plantar lateral position, thus respecting the joint's biomechanical axis. The first metatarsal is then reduced to close the intermetatarsal angle. Generally, there is a tendency to undercorrect the metatarsal plantarflexion. Too much dorsiflexion of the first ray may lead to transfer metatarsalgia of the second ray. If appropriate plantar-flexion cannot be achieved, the plantar lateral aspect of the joint should be revisualized to ensure that the joint is correctly prepared. It is relatively easy to leave residual cartilage or bony fragments on the plantar lateral of the joint aspect, which impede correct positioning. Local bone graft obtained from the medial MTP joint eminence may be placed into the arthrodesis site if there are any defects present. The correct alignment and rotation is fixed with a preliminary Kirschner wire. It is imperative that this checked both clinically and fluoroscopically.

Fixation with 2 crossed 3.5-mm lag screws is usually sufficient. A notch at the entry point of the distal screw prevents a fracture of the dorsal proximal cortex of the first metatarsal (**Fig. 2**). Without the notch, the screw levers the metatarsal cortex dorsally when cortical contact of the screw head forces it upwards. For the notch, a triangle of six 2.5-mm drill holes is created and the cortex surrounded by the drill holes is removed with a rongeur (**Fig. 3**). The medial cuneiform has a width of

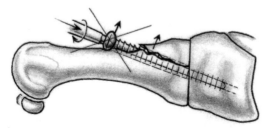

Fig. 2. A notch at the entry point of the distal screw prevents a fracture of the dorsal proximal cortex of the first metatarsal.

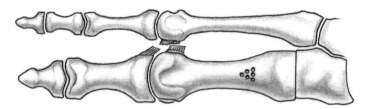

Fig. 3. For the notch, a triangle of six 2.5 mm drill holes is created and the cortex surrounded by the drill holes is removed with a rongeur.

approximately 1.5 cm. Appropriate aiming of the drill is crucial to correctly place the screws and to avoid violation of the intercuneiform joint. Drilling parallel to the medial border of the foot helps direct the drill in axis of the cuneiform. A 3.5-mm gliding hole is created. To allow more lateral correction of the first metatarsal, the 2.5-mm drill can then be directed in the cuneiform slightly more medially than the gliding hole (**Fig. 4**). A second screw is inserted from proximal to distal, aiming distally for the lateral plantar first metatarsal cortex. The screws should not cross within the fusion but rather distally to it, thus adding rotational stability. Dorsiflexion of the first MTPJ while inserting the screws improves compression at the arthrodesis site by tensioning the plantar fascia.

- The capsular tissues on the medial MTPJ are double-breasted for satisfactory alignment of the hallux. At this point, the deformity should be fully corrected. Any correction with dressings is not sufficient to prevent long-term recurrence. If there is residual deformity, the surgeon needs to ascertain the reason for this through clinical and flourscopic examination. Providing the arthrodesis has been fixed in the correct position, the most common reason is hallux interphalangeus. In this situation, an Akin osteotomy can be performed.
- The incision is then closed in layers. A compression dressing and a below-knee cast are applied.

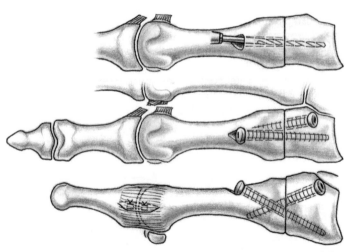

Fig. 4. A 3.5-mm gliding hole is created. To allow more lateral correction of the first metatarsal, the 2.5 mm drill can then be directed in the cuneiform slightly more medially than the gliding hole.

POSTOPERATIVE CARE

A compression dressing is removed 1 to 2 days after surgery and a below-knee cast is applied for 8 weeks. Patients are kept non–weight bearing for 4 weeks. The authors keep patients 10 to 20 kg partial weight bearing for the next 4 weeks.[24] Patients are then allowed transition to full weight bearing in regular shoes after this 8-week period of cast immobilization. In order to ensure progression of healing, the authors obtain dorsoplantar and lateral radiographs after 4 and 8 weeks.

Most investigators recommend non–weight bearing in the first 6 to 8 weeks after the procedure. Newer and stronger implants may provide more primary stability and, therefore, allow a shorter period of immobilization or immediate partial weight bearing postoperatively. Even full weight bearing 2 weeks after the procedure was described to have no adverse effects on alignment or the rate of osseous union.[25–27] Nevertheless, in biomechanical studies, most of these locking plates failed to demonstrate a stronger fixation than the crossed screw technique.[5,28–30] The downside of locking plates is the amount of hardware present in an area with little subcutaneous tissue. It is the authors' belief that locking plates have a greater potential for necessity of hardware removal. Even 2 crossed screws, however, cause implant-related problems in up to 20%.[31]

Because of the poor ratio of the long metatarsal lever arm and the small fusion surface, the authors do not recommend that patients be permitted to weight bear at an earlier stage. This cautiousness is supported by higher nonunion rates in several studies with early weight bearing as well as higher nonunion rates in simultaneous bilateral Lapidus fusion.[6,32]

Therefore, the classic construct of 2 crossed screws and an immobilization of 6 to 8 weeks still seems the gold standard. The authors' experience with this approach is generally good, and patients accept the longer period of cast immobilization and walking on crutches without complaints.

COMPLICATIONS AND MANAGEMENT

- The most common complication after a Lapidus procedure is nonunion. Rates from 2% to 10% are reported in the literature. In simultaneous bilateral operations, the rate even raises up to 33%.[6] Approximately 50% of the patients with nonunions are symptomatic and require revision.[33] Smoking is proved to have a major impact[11]; therefore, smoking is a relative contraindication for a Lapidus procedure in heavy smokers. Patients are informed about these risks and asked to stop or at least cut down smoking, but the authors do not cancel the surgery unless it is a revision surgery.

Table 2
Complications and management

Complications	Frequency (%)	Of Note
Nonunion	2–10[5,6,13,14,24,32,35,38–40]	Simultaneous bilateral operation: 33%[6] Symptomatic in 50%[33]
Transfer metatarsalgia	4–5[11,41]	Due to malalignment/shortening
Malunion	0–10[6,32,36]	
Hallux varus	0–16[39,40]	Mostly caused by excessive lateral release of the MTPJ 1
Recurrence	0–16[6,11,14,32,34,39,42]	

Table 3
Outcomes

Outcome	Rate/Range	Of Note
Reduction of HV angle	10°–22° [10,32,34,36,40]	
Reduction of IMT 1–2 angle	6°–9° [10,32,34,36,40]	
Patient satisfaction rate	74%–96% [3,5,32,34,42,43]	When performed after recurrence: 81% [11] Depending on [13] reduction of first intermetatarsal angle, first MTPJ dorsiflexion >45°, and proper sagittal alignment
Shortening of the first ray	2.9 mm–8 mm [6,11,13,37,41,44]	Management: 5–10 mm: plantarflexion of the first ray >10 mm: Weil osteotomies of second/ third ray >20 mm: lengthening with bone graft
Subjective foot stiffness	8%–18% [5,32,36]	
Prolonged pain/ swelling	Up to 16% [41]	Usually subsides after 3 mo

- In the presence of a painful nonunion, the authors recommend revision with autologous cancellous bone graft interposition and strong fixation, including fusion of the basis of the first and second metatarsals as originally described by Lapidus.
- Malalignment typically results in shortening and dorsiflexion of the first metatarsal and may lead to transfer metatarsalgia of the second and/or third rays. [14,34,35] It occurs in up to 10% of the cases. [36] It is, therefore, essential that accurate joint preparation is performed and that excessive wedges are not taken from the joint. Interposition of the resected medial eminence helps to prevent significant shortening if there is already a relatively short metatarsal or excessive bone has been resected. [37] A shortening of less than 5 mm with correct position usually does not cause problems. For shortening of 5 to 10 mm, a slight plantarflexion of the first metatarsal suffices to prevent problems. In cases of more than 10 mm, shortening metatarsal osteotomies (eg, Weil osteotomy) of the second and third toe can prevent transfer metatarsalgia. In cases of 20-mm and more first metatarsal shortening, however, a reconstruction of the first ray with a tricortical bone graft is used to adequately restore the correct length (**Tables 2 and 3**). [10]

SUMMARY

- The idea of the modified Lapidus procedure is to correct the hallux valgus where the primary deformity, the metatarsus primus varus, occurs.
- The Lapidus procedure is the most proximal site for forefoot correction and, therefore, offers more power than all metatarsal osteotomies.
- Accounting for 5% to 10% of all hallux valgus corrections, the modified Lapidus procedure is currently mainly used in severe deformities, deformity recurrences, first metatarsocuneiform arthritis, and hypermobility of the first ray.

- Because of its power and the demanding surgical technique, the procedure is prone to complications, which occur in approximately one-fourth of patients.
- With an appropriate surgical technique, good results can be expected, even when used for revision cases.
- Fixation with crossed screws and immobilization for 6 to 8 weeks still seem to be the gold standard.

REFERENCES

1. Albrecht GH. The pathology and treatment of hallux valgus. Russ Vrach 1911;10:14.
2. Truslow W. Metatarsus primus varus or hallux valgus? J Bone Joint Surg Am 1925; 7:98–108.
3. Kleinberg S. The operative cure of hallux valgus and bunions. Am J Surg 1932; 15:75–81.
4. Lapidus PW. Operative correction of the metatarsus varus primus in hallux valgus. Surg Gynecol Obstet 1934;58:16.
5. Clark HR, Veith RG, Hansen ST Jr. Adolescent bunions treated by the modified Lapidus procedure. Bull Hosp Jt Dis Orthop Inst 1987;47:109–22.
6. Sangeorzan BJ, Hansen ST Jr. Modified Lapidus procedure for hallux valgus. Foot Ankle 1989;9:262–6.
7. Morton DJ. The human foot. Columbia University Press; 1935.
8. Coughlin MJ, Jones CP. Hallux valgus: demographics, etiology, and radiographic assessment. Foot Ankle Int 2007;28:759–77.http://dx.doi.org/10.3113/FAI.2007.0759.
9. King DM, Toolan BC. Associated deformities and hypermobility in hallux valgus: an investigation with weightbearing radiographs. Foot Ankle Int 2004;25:251–5.
10. Coetzee JC, Resig SG, Kuskowski M, et al. The Lapidus procedure as salvage after failed surgical treatment of hallux valgus. Surgical technique. J Bone Joint Surg Am 2004;86A(Suppl 1):30–6.
11. Coetzee JC, Wickum D. The Lapidus procedure: a prospective cohort outcome study. Foot Ankle Int 2004;25:526–31.
12. Anderson M, Blais MM, Green WT. Lengths of the growing foot. J Bone Joint Surg Am 1956;38A:998–1000.
13. McInnes BD, Bouche RT. Critical evaluation of the modified Lapidus procedure. J Foot Ankle Surg 2001;40:71–90.
14. Catanzariti AR, Mendicino RW, Lee MS, et al. The modified Lapidus arthrodesis: a retrospective analysis. J Foot Ankle Surg 1999;38:322–32.
15. Glasoe WM, Allen MK, Ludewig PM. Comparison of first ray dorsal mobility among different forefoot alignments. J Orthop Sports Phys Ther 2000;30: 612–20 [discussion: 621–3].
16. Klaue K, Hansen ST, Masquelet AC. Clinical, quantitative assessment of first tarsometatarsal mobility in the sagittal plane and its relation to hallux valgus deformity. Foot Ankle Int 1994;15:9–13.
17. Beighton P, Solomon L, Soskolne CL. Articular mobility in an African population. Ann Rheum Dis 1973;32:413–8.
18. Grebing BR, Coughlin MJ. Evaluation of Morton's theory of second metatarsal hypertrophy. J Bone Joint Surg Am 2004;86A:1375–86.
19. Berntsen A. De l'hallux valgus: contribution a son etiologie et a son traitement. Rev Orthop 1930;3:101–11.
20. Ewald P. Die aetiologie des hallux valgus. Langenbecks Arch Surg 1912;114: 90–103.

21. Haines RW, McDougall A. The anatomy of hallux valgus. J Bone Joint Surg Br 1954;36B:272–93.
22. Mitchell CL, Fleming JL, Allen R, et al. Osteotomy-bunionectomy for hallux valgus. J Bone Joint Surg Am 1958;40A:41–58 [discussion: 59–60].
23. Myerson MS, Badekas A. Hypermobility of the first ray. Foot Ankle Clin 2000;5: 469–84.
24. Patel S, Ford LA, Etcheverry J, et al. Modified lapidus arthrodesis: rate of nonunion in 227 cases. J Foot Ankle Surg 2004;43:37–42.http://dx.doi.org/10. 1053/j.jfas.2003.11.009.
25. Basile P, Cook EA, Cook JJ. Immediate weight bearing following modified lapidus arthrodesis. J Foot Ankle Surg 2010;49:459–64.http://dx.doi.org/10.1053/j.jfas. 2010.06.003.
26. Blitz NM. Early weightbearing of the Lapidus bunionectomy: is it feasible? Clin Podiatr Med Surg 2012;29:367–81.http://dx.doi.org/10.1016/j.cpm.2012.04.009.
27. Cottom JM, Vora AM. Fixation of lapidus arthrodesis with a plantar interfragmentary screw and medial locking plate: a report of 88 cases. J Foot Ankle Surg 2013; 52:465–9.http://dx.doi.org/10.1053/j.jfas.2013.02.013.
28. Cohen DA, Parks BG, Schon LC. Screw fixation compared to H-locking plate fixation for first metatarsocuneiform arthrodesis: a biomechanical study. Foot Ankle Int 2005;26:984–9.
29. Egol KA, Kubiak EN, Fulkerson E, et al. Biomechanics of locked plates and screws. J Orthop Trauma 2004;18:488–93.
30. Johnson KA, Kile TA. Hallux valgus due to cuneiform-metatarsal instability. J South Orthop Assoc 1994;3:273–82.
31. Coetzee JC, Resig SG, Kuskowski M, et al. The Lapidus procedure as salvage after failed surgical treatment of hallux valgus: a prospective cohort study. J Bone Joint Surg Am 2003;85A:60–5.
32. Myerson M, Allon S, McGarvey W. Metatarsocuneiform arthrodesis for management of hallux valgus and metatarsus primus varus. Foot Ankle 1992;13: 107–15.
33. Thompson IM, Bohay DR, Anderson JG. Fusion rate of first tarsometatarsal arthrodesis in the modified Lapidus procedure and flatfoot reconstruction. Foot Ankle Int 2005;26:698–703.
34. Bednarz PA, Manoli A 2nd. Modified lapidus procedure for the treatment of hypermobile hallux valgus. Foot Ankle Int 2000;21:816–21.
35. Butson AR. A modification of the Lapidus operation for hallux valgus. J Bone Joint Surg Br 1980;62:350–2.
36. Myerson M. Metatarsocuneiform arthrodesis for treatment of hallux valgus and metatarsus primus varus. Orthopedics 1990;13:1025–31.
37. Fleming L, Savage TJ, Paden MH, et al. Results of modified lapidus arthrodesis procedure using medial eminence as an interpositional autograft. J Foot Ankle Surg 2011;50:272–5.http://dx.doi.org/10.1053/j.jfas.2011.02.012.
38. Grace D, Delmonte R, Catanzariti AR, et al. Modified lapidus arthrodesis for adolescent hallux abducto valgus. J Foot Ankle Surg 1999;38:8–13.
39. Kopp FJ, Patel MM, Levine DS, et al. The modified Lapidus procedure for hallux valgus: a clinical and radiographic analysis. Foot Ankle Int 2005;26:913–7.
40. Mauldin DM, Sanders M, Whitmer WW. Correction of hallux valgus with metatarsocuneiform stabilization. Foot Ankle 1990;11:59–66.
41. Rink-Brune O. Lapidus arthrodesis for management of hallux valgus–a retrospective review of 106 cases. J Foot Ankle Surg 2004;43:290–5.http://dx.doi.org/10. 1053/j.jfas.2004.07.007.

42. Lapidus PW. The author's bunion operation from 1931 to 1959. Clin Orthop 1960;
    16:119.
43. Goldner JL, Gaines RW. Adult and juvenile hallux valgus: analysis and treatment.
    Orthop Clin North Am 1976;7:863–87.
44. Lombardi CM, Silhanek AD, Connolly FG, et al. First metatarsocuneiform arthrod-
    esis and Reverdin-Laird osteotomy for treatment of hallux valgus: an
    intermediate-term retrospective outcomes study. J Foot Ankle Surg 2003;42:
    77–85.http://dx.doi.org/10.1053/jfas.2003.50014.

Pediatric Hallux Valgus

Julian Chell, MBBS, FRCS(Orth),
Sunil Dhar, MBBS, MS, MCh Orth, FRCS(Ed Orth)*

KEYWORDS

- Childhood hallux valgus • Open physes • Orthotics and braces
- Surgical intervention

KEY POINTS

- The treating surgeon should be aware of the varying anatomic relationships that can occur in adolescent hallux valgus, and assessment of these is crucial when analyzing each individual's presentation so that definitive treatment is tailored to that individual, to correct the underlying deformity and achieve long-term correction.
- The role of surgical correction in children with open physes is limited, and should be delayed until skeletal maturity.

INTRODUCTION

Hallux valgus in children is a relatively uncommon deformity, also known by several other names such as juvenile or adolescent bunion, metatarsus primus varus, and metatarsus primus adductus. Although there is no agreed precise definition of pediatric hallux valgus, the presence of an open growth plate is considered by most to be part of the definition of this condition. However, others include patients up to age 20 years, owing to the plastic nature of the various components of the condition.

The presenting complaint is invariably of the bunion and its cosmetic appearance. Occasionally, pain may be the predominant symptom.

PATHOGENESIS

The pathogenesis of hallux valgus is complex, and there can be multiple variations in the underlying anatomy. More than 80% of children presenting with this condition will be female and approximately half of these will present before the age of 10 years. Maternal transmission is common, particularly in those younger than 10 years at presentation.[1] It is estimated that 40% to 50% of adult bunions actually have their onset in childhood.

Department of Orthopaedics, Nottingham University Hospitals, City Hospital Campus, Nottingham NG5 1PB, UK
* Corresponding author.
E-mail address: sunil.dahr@btinternet.com

Foot Ankle Clin N Am 19 (2014) 235–243
http://dx.doi.org/10.1016/j.fcl.2014.02.007
1083-7515/14/$ – see front matter © 2014 Elsevier Inc. All rights reserved.

The etiologic basis for the pathologic deformity is considered to be metatarsus primus varus, which has been detected in infancy,[1–3] but there often are other anatomic abnormalities present. There may be an oblique first metatarsal–cuneiform articulation. The distal metatarsal articular angle (DMAA) can be laterally deviated, which invariably occurs in those younger than 10 years,[1] and the first metatarsophalangeal joint (MTPJ) may be flat or conical.

Hallux valgus is also said to be associated with flexible pes planus and ligamentous laxity, although this is prevalent in this population in any event, and some investigators have noted no increase in its presence in comparison with the normal population.[1,2] The first metatarsal may be long, which is associated with an increase in the DMAA,[1] and the first ray may be hypermobile.

As the hallux valgus increases, typically the great toe pronates and the sesamoids begin to be carried laterally by the short flexor and adductor tendons. The medial soft tissues become stretched and the pronation causes the abductor hallucis to be moved in a plantar direction, negating its normal counterbalancing effect on the adductor, and together with ligamentous laxity results in splaying of the foot.[1,2] Flexible pes planus causing pronation of the forefoot will further worsen the changes that occur as hallux valgus progresses: the great toe is pronated and therefore the abductor hallucis is in a more plantar position, hence the imbalance around the MTPJ occurs.[1,2]

Metatarsus adductus is often present, with rates being on the order of 1:5. However, this is not associated with increased deformity or a change in surgical correction techniques, or their success.[1]

Shoe wear per se is not a cause of the deformity, although more likely than not it is a cause of symptoms.[3]

The deformity is also associated with other neuromuscular conditions such as cerebral palsy, when muscle overactivity may be the sole cause of the deformity and there will be minimal bony abnormality.[4]

Hallux interphalangeus is commonly associated with hallux valgus, and needs careful clinical and radiologic assessment in considering its presence and the need for correction as a combined procedure.[1,3]

INVESTIGATION AND ASSESSMENT

A full and thorough examination of the foot and ankle is necessary to assess for the presence of a flat-foot deformity and whether this is flexible or rigid. The presence of callosities that indicate transfer metatarsalgia should be noted. The hallux valgus deformity should be assessed and noted as to whether this is passively correctable, and the foot position and width noted with correction being achieved. Other associated deformities such as hallux interphalangeus and metatarsus adductus should be recognized.

Assessment by radiologic investigation is essential by formal weight-bearing anteroposterior and lateral views of the feet, with non–weight-bearing oblique views. Radiography allows full appreciation of the underlying deformity and accurate measurement of the hallux valgus angle, the intermetatarsal angle, the inclination of the metatarsal-cuneiform articulation, and the DMAA, so that a formal treatment plan can be decided upon to correct any abnormalities present (**Fig. 1**).

The inclination of the metatarsocuneiform joint is taken in relation to the longitudinal axis of the foot. It should also be noted as to whether there is an articular facet at this level between the first and second metatarsals, as this will restrict corrections at that level (ie, a metatarsocuneiform fusion).

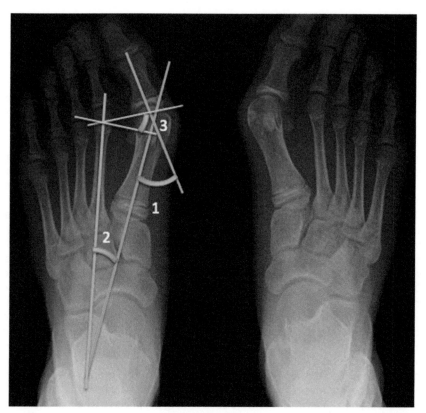

Fig. 1. The hallux valgus angle is the angle subtended by a line drawn along the central longitudinal axis of the first metatarsal and a second line drawn along the central longitudinal axis of the proximal phalanx (1). The intermetatarsal angle is the angle subtended at the intersection of 2 lines drawn along the central axes of the first and second metatarsals (2). The distal metatarsal articular angle is the angle subtended by a line drawn parallel to the articular surface and the central longitudinal axis line of the first metatarsal (3).

The congruence of the first MTPJ should be noted, as it is considered that a congruent joint is stable whereas an incongruent joint has become unstable and, therefore, the hallux valgus deformity is likely to progress.[3]

Radiographs also allow assessment of the epiphyseal plates and whether growth has finished, because being variable this may be used to advise on timing with regard to surgical intervention, as recurrence rates are higher when growth is still active.

In the presence of a rigid flat-foot deformity, further investigation may be required if the oblique views of the foot do not demonstrate a calcaneonavicular coalition, and a computed tomography scan to exclude other coalitions may be required. Forefoot corrections will be compromised by the presence of a rigid flat-foot deformity, and one needs to consider management of this as either a combined or a staged procedure.[1,2]

Mild deformities are generally defined as those with an intermetatarsal angle greater than 10° and a hallux valgus angle greater than 20°. Moderate deformities are with a hallux valgus angle of 25° to 40° and severe deformities are those with a hallux valgus angle greater than 40°.[1–3]

CONSERVATIVE MANAGEMENT

Timing of operative intervention should, wherever possible, be at or beyond skeletal maturity,[1,2] to allow time for the completion of growth and, hence, possibly prevent recurrence or overcorrection as a result. It also allows time for the soft tissues to mature, ligamentous laxity will often naturally reduce, and any associated flexible pes planus has time to improve, all of which are useful counseling points to both parents and the adolescent when delaying the time of intervention to a time point with a higher success rate.

Delaying the procedure does mean that the deformity will have had the chance to progress, so the surgical technique to correct the deformity may eventually be more extensive than required at first presentation. This risk needs to be balanced against the risk of recurrence, and therefore the risk of early revision surgery if surgery is performed when the patient is skeletally immature.

The authors recommend that before skeletal maturity, treatment should be conservative wherever possible. If the deformity is asymptomatic, no intervention is required. Parents and patients should be advised to watch for onset of symptoms and progression of deformity, and to review as required. When symptoms are present, basic advice with regard to shoewear and activity modification may be all that is required.

Orthotic input is useful when there is a painful bunion associated with flexible pes planus, because stabilization of the latter often helps the bunion pain experienced, although care has to be taken that this does not increase the pressure on the area of the exostoses, thereby increasing pain in this region from footwear.[5,6] Bracing can also be used, although one has to advise that this will not provide long-term correction but can be a useful means of symptomatic relief.

In one study, nighttime splintage combined with passive and active exercise regimes achieved improvement in the intermetatarsal angle and the MTPJ angle in 50% of cases, and no recurrences were seen among the patients who had improved.[6]

Bracing has not been shown to prevent the progression of radiologic changes associated with hallux valgus deformity, nor does it prevent the development of this condition. In cases where patients presented with unilateral hallux valgus despite the use of bilateral bracing, hallux valgus still developed on the initially unaffected side.[5]

It is the authors' experience, however, that because the major presenting population is adolescent girls bracing is often not well tolerated, being considered cumbersome in shoewear and unsightly in nature. It is therefore uncommon that most patients will wear the braces provided.

OPERATIVE INTERVENTION

The indication for operation is essentially pain; however, the form and timing of the procedure are more difficult. The degree of the deformity is not in itself an indication for treatment, and symptom severity often does not reflect the degree of clinical or radiologic change present.

Operative intervention requires careful planning because bony realignment is the key to a successful outcome, and reliance on soft-tissue correction is often met with early recurrence owing to the general laxity and elasticity of these tissues.[1,2]

More than 130 different procedures have been described for the management of this condition, which fall into 4 basic categories: proximal metatarsal osteotomy, distal metatarsal osteotomy, soft-tissue procedures, and combined procedures.[2]

There is no singular superior treatment option, nor one that is specific to any particular group of patients, but there are some general principles to be followed.

If surgery is to be performed before closure of the epiphyseal plates, the treatment options are more limited if compromise of the physes is to be avoided. Proximal metatarsal osteotomies are generally described in the area of the growth plate, as are proximal phalangeal osteotomies; therefore, these are generally contraindicated. There is the attraction of a distal metatarsal osteotomy, although this is limited with regard to correction if there is a large deformity. It can be challenging to address all underlying abnormalities, such as variations in the DMAA, with a distal osteotomy. If there is still a considerable period of growth left, the first metatarsal with metatarsus primus varus will continue to grow in an abnormal alignment, compromising long-term results. Therefore, for those children in whom growth remains and who have failed conservative management, alternative techniques should be considered.

Simple bunionectomy can be performed in cases where the pain is related to pressure alone, acknowledging to the patient and family that this is not going to correct the underlying deformity. It is also necessary to explain that the deformity is likely to recur but, where the pain is specific and it can be accepted that this is only a temporizing measure, it is not an unreasonable procedure before formal bony correction. It is the authors' experience that while in theory this seems acceptable, it is rarely the case that sufficient relief occurs or, when it does, it is for insufficient time before symptoms recur.

A more attractive proposition is put forward by combining removal of the bunion with more extensive soft-tissue procedures including release or transfer of the adductor hallucis, a lateral capsular release, and medial capsule placation, which can also be combined with excision of the fibular sesamoid, the modified McBride procedures. These techniques are often considered more physiologic in nature and have been reported as having considerable success, although the most concerning complication is of hallux varus, which is associated with more extensive corrections and younger individuals.[7] Because of the risk of developing hallux varus, the authors do not recommend a lateral sesamoidectomy.

The treatment regime recommended by Coughlin[1] is noteworthy. The degree of the deformity was assessed and the operative intervention planned accordingly, so that for mild deformities a chevron osteotomy or a McBride procedure (but avoiding a lateral sesamoidectomy) was undertaken; for increased deformities with MTPJ subluxation a distal soft-tissue correction and a proximal osteotomy, distal to the physis, was performed, and for increased deformities with an increased DMAA, combined double osteotomies were undertaken. This regime gave a good or excellent result in 92% of cases.

Distal metatarsal osteotomies such as a Mitchell osteotomy have been extensively reported with varying results, which may reflect variations in operative technique. Improved results have been noted with internal fixation or when a more stable configuration of osteotomy, such as a chevron, has been used.[8–10] Distal metatarsal osteotomies do create an element of metatarsal shortening, and therefore will be useful in the correction of juvenile hallux valgus associated with a long first metatarsal. In principle, however, they are not as assured in altering the DMAA, and this deformity is typically associated with a long first metatarsal. In the authors' opinion, these osteotomies are suitable for mild deformities at skeletal maturity whereby the intermetatarsal angle is not significantly increased and there is no significant increase in the DMAA.

For mild or moderate deformities whereby there is an increase in the DMAA, techniques such as the scarf osteotomy allow for better correction (**Fig. 2**). This method will maintain metatarsal length or allow shortening if necessary if the first metatarsal is overly long, but at the same time rotation can be undertaken to correct the DMAA to within the normal range, which is considered beneficial to a successful outcome.

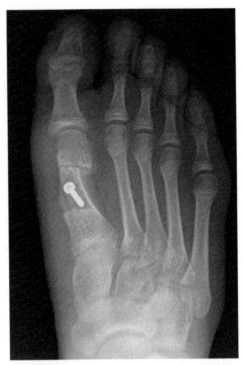

Fig. 2. Scarf osteotomy to correct hallux valgus in a 12-year-old patient (same patient as in **Fig. 1**) 7 months postoperatively. The outcome was satisfactory, with a congruent joint and correction of deformity.

When there is evidence of instability or hypermobility at the first tarsometatarsal joint with a significant hallux valgus deformity, consideration of fusion of this joint (the Lapidus procedure) will help to achieve stability, and allows correction of the deformity in a manner similar to that of a proximal metatarsal osteotomy. The Lapidus procedure was actually developed as a means of treating metatarsus primus varus, and it has been postulated that part of the reason for this is the angulation of the metatarsocuneiform joint and the relative hypermobility of children causing increased mobility in that area. Therefore, fusion stabilizes the joint and addresses the abnormal area.[11] However, it does not address any associated distal abnormality, although it may be combined with other procedures to fully address the abnormalities present. It is clear that waiting for skeletal maturity is mandatory before performing the fusion. However, in the uncommon instance of an unstable first metatarsocuneiform joint and an unduly long first metatarsal in a child with open physes, a Lapidus procedure may be beneficial. Of course the potential remaining growth must be taken into consideration.

OUTCOMES OF SURGERY

Recurrence rates are age dependent, and there is an increased recurrence rate for those who are skeletally immature.

For the modified McBride procedures in a series of 17 feet it was stated that the outcome was good in 10, satisfactory in 2, and dissatisfying in 5 at an average 14-year follow-up.[7]

In 1995 Coughlin[1] reported 45 patients (60 feet) with a recurrence rate of 6 feet (10%) over an 11-year period.

For distal metatarsal osteotomies such as the Mitchell osteotomy, recurrence rates of up to 61%[12] have been reported, although others have reported successful correction in up to 95%.[13] In part this may reflect the patient population and lack of fixation of the osteotomy.

Proximal crescentic operations have been noted to maintain metatarsal length and result in a good outcome.[14] Dome osteotomies may worsen the DMAA, which may affect outcome, although success rates of more than 80% are reported.[14] Wedge osteotomies have been reported to have poorer outcomes. Opening wedge osteotomies have been noted to have a higher recurrence rate,[15] and closing wedge osteotomies are associated with shortening and metatarsalgia.[16]

The Lapidus procedure also has been used in adolescent hallux valgus.[11,17] In a series of 30 feet, good or excellent results were reported in 27 feet (90%); however, the age range of patients was 13 to 20 years.[11] Similarly in the series by Clark and colleagues,[17] the average age of the patients was older than 18 years. The authors believe that this procedure should be limited to patients who are skeletally mature.

The results of scarf osteotomy in children are more promising,[18–21] though conflicting. John and colleagues[18] reported on 7 patients who had the procedure at an average age of 14 years, with only 1 recurrence after 14 years. Farrar and colleagues[19] reported 93% satisfactory results at 3 years in 39 feet treated with the scarf osteotomy at a mean age of 14 years. Young and colleagues[20] reported satisfactory results in 16 feet, although the mean age of the patients was 22 years (ie, adults). However, George and colleagues[21] found an unacceptable recurrence rate in 19 feet operated on at a mean age of 14 years, and cautioned against the use of scarf osteotomy.

PATHOLOGIC HALLUX VALGUS

In neurologic conditions such as cerebral palsy, hallux valgus can often present and is progressive in nature, and deformity can be extreme. In this situation, while there can be similar underlying anatomic abnormalities to the bony structures as in non-neurologic hallux valgus, the deformity is more often related to the high muscle tone.

Assessment is as for idiopathic hallux valgus, and the main aim of treatment is to provide a stable, comfortable position of the great toe that is pain free. Radiologic examination is useful when considering the possibility of other underlying abnormalities and to exclude allied conditions. However, these often have little bearing on the treatment.

In the growing child with open growth plates, purely conservative treatment is recommended by way of orthoses and shoewear modification until the end of growth, and treatment should be deferred until this time. The indication for surgical intervention is symptomatic hallux valgus affecting gait and shoewear, and the preferred option is by fusion of the first MTPJ. This option gives the greatest degree of correction and the best outcome when compared with other techniques.[22] All other forms of intervention to treat this condition along the treatment lines of idiopathic hallux valgus lead to a much greater rate of recurrence because of the underlying muscle imbalance that cannot be corrected by balancing of soft tissues. First MTPJ fusion provides a stable great toe in a physiologic alignment and allows mobility to be maintained, without the concerns of recurrence. It has also been shown to achieve high reports of carer satisfaction with regard to cosmesis, footwear, hygiene, activity levels, and pain, and is the treatment of choice in this situation.[4]

SUMMARY

The treating surgeon should be aware of the varying anatomic relationships that can occur in adolescent hallux valgus, and assessment of these is crucial when analyzing each individual's presentation so that definitive treatment is tailored to that individual, to correct the underlying deformity and achieve long-term correction. The role of surgical correction in children with open physes is limited, and should be delayed until skeletal maturity.

REFERENCES

1. Coughlin MJ. Roger A. Mann Award. Juvenile hallux valgus: etiology and treatment. Foot Ankle Int 1995;16(11):682–97.
2. Herring A. Tachdjian's pediatric orthopaedics. 3rd edition. Philadelphia: WB Saunders; 2002. p. 1012–37.
3. Tachdjian MO. Clinical pediatric orthopaedics: the art of diagnosis and the principles of management. Stamford (CT): Appleton & Lange; 1997. p. 55–9.
4. Davids JR, Mason TA, Danko A, et al. Surgical management of hallux valgus deformity in children with cerebral palsy. J Pediatr Orthop 2001;21(1):89–94.
5. Kilmartin TE, Barrington RL, Wallace WA. A controlled prospective trial of a foot orthosis for juvenile hallux valgus. J Bone Joint Surg Br 1994;76(2):210–4.
6. Groiso JA. Juvenile hallux valgus. A conservative approach to treatment. J Bone Joint Surg Am 1992;74(9):1367–74.
7. Schwillate M, Karbowski A, Eckhardt A. Hallux valgus in young patients: long-term results after McBride operation. Arch Orthop Trauma Surg 1997;116(6–7): 412–4.
8. Zimmer TJ, Johnson KA, Klassen RA. Treatment of hallux valgus in adolescents by Chevron osteotomy. Foot Ankle 1989;9:190–3.
9. Das De S. Distal metatarsal osteotomy for adolescent hallux valgus. J Pediatr Orthop 1984;1:32–8.
10. Luba R, Rosman M. Bunions in children: treatment with a modified Mitchell osteotomy. J Pediatr Orthop 1984;4A:44–7.
11. Grace D, Delmonte R, Catanzariti AR, et al. Modified Lapidus arthrodesis for adolescent hallux abducto valgus. J Foot Ankle Surg 1999;38:8–13.
12. Ball J, Sullivan J. Treatment of juvenile bunion by the Mitchell osteotomy. Orthopedics 1985;18:1249–52.
13. Geissele AE, Stanton RP. Surgical treatment of adolescent hallux valgus. J Pediatr Orthop 1990;10A:642–8.
14. Petratos D, Anastasopoulos J, Plakogiannis C, et al. Correction of adolescent hallux valgus by proximal crescentic osteotomy of the first metatarsal. Acta Orthop Belg 2008;74:496–502.
15. Thodarson DB, Leventen EO. Hallux valgus correction with proximal metatarsal osteotomy: two year follow-up. Foot Ankle 1992;13:321–6.
16. Resch S, Strentrom A, Egund N. Proximal closing wedge osteotomy and adductor tenotomy for treatment of hallux valgus. Foot Ankle 1989;9:272–80.
17. Clark HR, Veith RG, Hansen ST Jr. Adolescent bunions treated by the modified Lapidus procedure. Bull Hosp Jt Dis Orthop Inst 1987;47(2):109–22.
18. John S, Weil L Jr, Weil LS Sr, et al. Scarf osteotomy for the correction of adolescent hallux valgus. Foot Ankle Spec 2010;3(1):10–4.
19. Farrar NG, Duncan N, Ahmed N, et al. Scarf osteotomy in the management of symptomatic adolescent hallux valgus. J Child Orthop 2012;6(2):153–7.

20. Young KW, Kim JS, Cho JW, et al. Characteristics of male adolescent-onset hallux valgus. Foot Ankle Int 2013;34(8):1111–6.
21. George HL, Casaletto J, Unnikrishnan PN, et al. Outcome of the scarf osteotomy in adolescent hallux valgus. J Child Orthop 2009;3(3):185–90.
22. Jenter M, Lipton GE, Miller F. Operative treatment for hallux valgus in children with cerebral palsy. Foot Ankle Int 1998;19(12):830–5.

First Metatarsophalangeal Arthrodesis for Hallux Valgus

Edward V. Wood, FRCS(Tr&Orth)[a],*,
Christopher R. Walker, MCH(Orth), FRCS(Orth), FRCS(Eng), FRCS(Ed)[b],
Michael S. Hennessy, BSc, FRCSEd(Tr&Orth)[c]

KEYWORDS

- Hallux • Valgus • Arthrodesis • Fusion • Metatarsophalangeal

KEY POINTS

- Arthrodesis of the first metatarsophalangeal joint reliably improves the deformity of both hallux valgus (HV) and metatarsus primus varus.
- This technique is well suited to patients with an irritable or degenerate first metatarsophalangeal joint, those with a severe deformity, HV associated with inflammatory arthritis and patients of advanced age.
- Failed primary HV surgery can be reliably salvaged using an arthrodesis of the first metatarsophalangeal joint.

INTRODUCTION

Arthrodesis of the first metatarsophalangeal (MTP) joint is a reliable operation in the treatment of selected cases of hallux valgus (HV). Not only does it correct the HV, but the metatarsus primus varus deformity is also addressed. It is an operation with good functional results and a low complication rate. This technique is most appropriate for patients with HV associated with degenerative changes or severe deformity, and those for whom primary HV surgery has failed.

PATHOGENESIS OF HALLUX VALGUS

The pathogenesis of HV has previously been well described, and for an in-depth description the reader is directed to the article by Perera and colleagues,[1] and

Conflicts of Interest: None of the authors has any relationships with a commercial company that has a direct financial interest in the subject matter or materials discussed in this article, or with a company making a competing product.
[a] Department of Orthopaedics, Countess of Chester Hospital NHS Trust, Liverpool Road, Chester CH2 1UL, UK; [b] Department of Orthopaedics, Royal Liverpool University Hospital, Prescot Street, Liverpool L7 8XP, UK; [c] Department of Orthopaedics, Wirral University Hospitals NHS Trust, Arrowe Park Road, Upton, Wirral CH49 5PE, UK
* Corresponding author.
E-mail address: edward.wood@nhs.net

additional studies by Coughlin[2] and Shereff.[3] The anatomy of the hallux and first metatarsal is also well described in the anatomic study by Scranton and Rutkowski.[4]

The fundamental steps are as follows:

- Failure of the medial structures (tibial sesamoid and medial collateral ligaments)
- Medial displacement of the first metatarsal head, with subluxation of the sesamoid apparatus
- The hallux is drawn into a valgus position by the effect of the deep transverse ligament and adductor hallucis, which also pulls the hallux into pronation because of its plantar attachment
- The long flexor and extensor tendons act as bowstrings, further increasing the HV
- The abductor hallucis becomes dysfunctional as its insertion rotates toward the plantar aspect

INDICATIONS

The indications for surgery in HV are accepted as pain, secondary to the deformity, which is refractory to nonoperative measures. The difficulty in decision making lies in knowing when to use joint-conserving techniques or when to use an arthrodesis. Several indications for arthrodesis have been proposed:

- Failed HV surgery (recurrent deformity, hallux varus, or avascular necrosis)[5,6]
- Severe HV deformity[5–7]
- HV secondary to neuromuscular disorders[5,6]
- Rheumatoid arthritis[5,6,8,9]
- HV in advanced age[10]
- Arthritis secondary to infection (resolved)[2,11]
- HV with degenerative joint disease[7]
- Moderate to severe HV associated with metatarsalgia[6]

Investigators have proposed treatment algorithms. In Coughlin and colleagues'[6] series of 21 fusions for HV the indications were moderate HV (angle 21°–40°) with secondary degenerative changes or medial column instability, or all severe HV (>40°) (**Table 1**).

There may be merit in bias toward joint-conserving surgery; in a comparison between Scarf osteotomy and first MTP joint fusion, although there was no difference in terms of pain, complications, and global satisfaction, the Scarf group showed superior results in terms of functional outcome, particularly reflected in the Foot and Ankle Ability Measure (FAAM) scores.[12] However, the indications and preoperative clinical features of the groups were not specified, and it is recognized that the pathologic characteristics of the 2 groups was different.[12]

Assessment of irritability of the first MTP joint is also important, as the degree of osteoarthritis is underestimated on plain films. This evaluation is undertaken clinically

Table 1 Classification of hallux valgus		
Classification	Hallux Valgus Angle	Intermetatarsal Angle
Normal	<15°	<9°
Mild	15°–20°	<11°
Moderate	20°–40°	11°–16°
Severe	>40°	>16°

Modified from Coughlin MJ. Hallux valgus. J Bone Joint Surg Am 1996;78(6):932–66.

using the axial grind test with the hallux in the corrected position. The severity of deformity should influence decision making; as the deformity increases, so does the severity of the cartilage lesions found within the joint.[13]

It is difficult to be prescriptive regarding the indications for fusion in HV, but the authors consider that the aforementioned approach by Coughlin is reasonable. Ultimately it is a decision formed by discussion with the patient and informed by one's own clinical judgment.

EVOLUTION OF THE SURGICAL TECHNIQUE

The aim of surgery is to relieve pain, restore comfortable gait, correct deformity, and, in doing so, improve shoe fit. Many techniques have been described, and it is beyond the scope of this article to discuss these in detail. The main choices lie in the preparation of the joint surfaces and the method of fixation. Regarding the former, planar cuts, peg-and-socket techniques, or more spherical cup-and-cone techniques have been described in the literature. Planar cuts have the advantage of being quick but, if repositioning is required, further cuts lead to loss of bone stock and shortening.[14] Peg-and-socket techniques have the advantage of inherent stability but lose bone stock, cause shortening, and are technically demanding.[15–18] Hemispherical cup-and-cone techniques have the advantage of being easily and reproducibly performed with cannulated reamers.[14] These methods allow intraoperative repositioning, in all planes, without further bone loss, provide a large surface area for union, and have been shown to be biomechanically superior to planar cuts when fixation is applied.[19,20]

Regarding fixation techniques, compressive internal fixation has become the norm. This technique may involve screws, plates, or a combination of the two, and more recently the use of memory staples has also been described.[10,11,14,17,18,21–27] Biomechanical studies of fixation techniques have shown that a dorsal plate combined with an interfragmentary lag screw provides the most stable fixation in comparison with isolated plate, screw, or Kirschner (K)-wire fixation.[28,29] This finding is reflected in the standard technique used by the authors: preparation of the joint surfaces using cup-and-cone reamers, stabilized with a contoured dorsal plate and an interfragmentary screw.

PLATE DESIGN

Specifically designed, precontoured plates prevent excessive dorsiflexion and may help prevent failure seen with generic plates that need to be bent, and therefore weakened, at the time of procedure.[30] Locking-plate technology is now becoming widely accepted owing to several practical and perceived superior mechanical properties. This technology was developed particularly for fracture fixation in osteoporotic bone and periarticular fractures, and provides a useful adjunct in forefoot surgery. The theoretical advantage of superior construct rigidity has led to a subsequent explosion in the use of locking plates in the foot. However, in a recent study comparing locked and nonlocked fixation in MTP arthrodesis, the union rate in the nonlocked group was actually higher than that in the locked-plate group.[31] This finding suggests that locked plates may not provide the same perceived advantages in this scenario. Hence it is vital that proper biomechanical data and full clinical outcomes/trial results are available before such implants are given general approval, thus allowing clinicians to both confirm and optimize the indications for their use. Hunt and colleagues[32] performed an in vitro biomechanical study to explain the previous results. This group compared load to failure tests in 2 groups of cadaveric specimens (9 matched pairs), prepared with cup-and-cone reamers, with fixation of the MTP joint with a compression screw and either a nonlocked or locked stainless-steel dorsal plate. The locked-plate group demonstrated less plantar gapping in fatigue endurance, and there was greater stiffness in the locked-plate construct. In this study it is clear that compression-screw fixation was performed before the application of either the locked or nonlocked plates (the correct technique in the view of the authors). In the earlier study by Hunt and colleagues[31] the MTP joint was provisionally fixed with a K-wire, followed by dorsal plate positioning using K-wires and then placement of an interfragmentary screw. The plate was then secured with screws. It is possible that the wire fixation of the plate may have compromised the compression obtained by the lag screw, thus giving rise to the somewhat paradoxic higher nonunion rate in the locked-plate group because of "a diminished ability to obtain sufficient inter-fragmentary compression with the locked-plate design and the inferior rigidity of the titanium plate compared to the stainless steel plate."[31] It is also possible that the difference may be due to the use, or not, of a lag screw, although this is difficult to determine from the article. In their biomechanical study, however, there was no statistically significant difference in ultimate load to failure between the 2 methods of fixation. Failure in the locked-plate group tended to be by bone fracture and that in the nonlocked group by plate bending, thus reflecting the differences in mean stiffness between the groups. The investigators concluded that "it is possible that locked plates produce an environment that is too stiff to reliably promote bone healing if there is not sufficient compression and bony contact at the time of plate application."[32] This finding is supported by other literature on the subject of locked plates, which suggests that interfragmentary motion may be suppressed to a level not conducive to bone healing[33]; this also reflects the accepted truism that in any fusion procedure, there is a race between bone healing and hardware failure on weight bearing.

On its own, a low-profile plate cannot provide sufficient rigidity to reliably promote fusion. Compression remains the best method of ensuring stability. A dorsal plate is on the compressive surface of the first MTP joint, so an interfragmentary lag screw is important in preventing opening of the plantar aspect of the joint on weight bearing. If locking plates are used alone, a higher nonunion rate should be expected. Although compression can be achieved by the surgeon squeezing the surfaces together, or through the use of a compressive hole in the plate, the authors believe that compression using a lag screw, neutralized with a dorsal plate, is the more reliable technique.

MECHANISM OF CORRECTION

The bunion deformity comprises 2 main elements: HV and metatarsus primus varus. The HV deformity is, in part, caused by the action of the adductor inserting to the base of the proximal phalanx via the conjoined tendon. Therefore if the adductor is maintained, repositioning the metatarsal head beneath the base of the proximal phalanx will reduce the deformity. The metatarsus primus varus deformity is also addressed by fusion of the first MTP joint with narrowing of the intermetatarsal angle (IMA). For this to occur, the first metatarsocuneiform joint needs to be mobile and the adductor tendon needs to be intact. Through its attachment to the base of the proximal phalanx, the adductor now acts as a check-rein or anchor point on which the metatarsal can be reduced. The arthrodesis/fixation then maintains the relationship between the first metatarsal and the hallux. Through this the adductor now acts on the first metatarsal, pulling it toward the midline and thus reducing the IMA.[14] Thus the action of the adductor changes from a deforming force to a corrective force (**Figs. 1** and **2**).

With correction of the position of the first metatarsal, the stability of the medial column is restored. This stability allows increased medial column weight bearing which, in turn, reduces lateral or transfer metatarsalgia.[6,9,15,18,23]

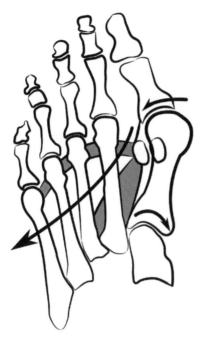

Fig. 1. Adductor generates hallux valgus deformity.

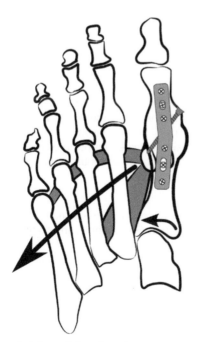

Fig. 2. Adductor now corrects intermetatarsal angle.

Hallux Valgus Correction

Arthrodesis of the first MTP joint can be considered a reliable technique for correction of the HV deformity. Moderate deformities can be corrected to normal, as shown in separate studies by Riggs and Johnson[34] and Pydah and colleagues[35]: the mean preoperative HV angles were 35° and 33°, correcting to 14° and 10.4°, respectively (see **Table 1**). Where the deformity is graded as severe, the final correction may not return to normal but correct to "mild"; Tourné and colleagues[10] reported a mean preoperative HV angle of 43° correcting to 17°. In Coughlin's[9] series of first MTP joint fusions for rheumatoid arthritis, the mean preoperative HV angle was 38° correcting to 20°. By contrast, however, Mann and Katcherian[25] showed no correlation between the severity of the IMA on the ability to correct the HV angle, and in their series obtained HV corrections to 12.6°.

Intermetatarsal Angle Correction

Numerous investigators have shown a reduction of the IMA of between 3.0° and 8.2° from the preoperative values.[6,9,10,16,25,34–38] Along with this there is a concomitant reduction in the width of the foot: Raymakers and Waugh[23] noted an average reduction in foot width of 6 mm, ascribing this to "improved muscle function," and later Coughlin and colleagues[6] noted a mean narrowing of the foot of 9.0 mm following fusion.

Severity of IMA

In their 1989 series, Mann and Katcherian[25] showed that the group with the largest IMA also had the greatest correction: those with an IMA of at least 19° had a mean correction of 8.8°, those with an IMA of 13° or greater had a mean correction of 6.6°, and those with an IMA of 12° or less had a mean correction of only 2.4°.[25] In another series, Cronin and colleagues[36] also showed a greater correction with increasing deformity, with a mean correction of the IMA of 6.1° in those with a preoperative IMA of 15° or less, and a correction of 9.9° in those with a preoperative IMA of at least 16°. Pydah and colleagues[35] again showed similar findings, but there was no difference in the magnitude of correction between the moderate and severe groups, which showed a correction of 7.1° and 6.8°, respectively. Sung and colleagues[37] also showed a larger correction with increasing severity of IMA, but the final IMA remained greater as the severity of the preoperative deformity increased. Those with a mild IMA corrected to within normal limits (10.0°–8.3°), whereas those with a severe deformity corrected to a moderate IMA (18.1°–11.4°).[37] Several investigators conclude that the degree of correction of the IMA by fusion obviates further proximal procedures.[6,25,35,38] It has also been noted that the IMA may also continue to reduce with time.[16]

OPERATIVE TECHNIQUE

The precise technique will vary according to the primary abnormality, anatomy, and any other procedures being performed. For example, any significant hallux interphalangeus deformity necessitates eccentric bone resection of the proximal phalanx with more bone removed medially to correct the overall alignment. Consideration must also be given to the shortening that may be necessary in severe deformity to achieve correction because of chronic soft-tissue contracture. The authors prefer not to remove all subchondral bone, as this confers some structural stability. However, if there is a severe deformity some shortening will be necessary and, hence, the subchondral bone will need to be resected. In osteoporotic patients or those with rheumatoid disease the bone is often of poor quality, and care should be taken not to over-ream.

Incision

A dorsal midline approach is favored, the advantage here being access to the joint, ease of positioning of the fusion, and hardware placement. However, if the fusion is one of several forefoot procedures being performed (especially in patients with multiple abnormality/deformity, eg, rheumatoid), a medial incision can be used to maintain a reasonable "skin bridge." To use the adductor to correct the IMA, no attempt is made to release the lateral structures.[35,36]

Joint Preparation

The authors prepare the joint in a standard fashion, removing larger osteophytes with osteotomes and nibblers, and use hemispherical, cup-and-cone reamers to remove the articular surfaces to bleeding subchondral bone. The reamed surfaces are then breached multiple times with a 1.6-mm K-wire.

Positioning and Fixation

There are many references regarding the ideal position of the great toe relative to age, gender, and foot type. The authors recommend positioning of the phalanx relative to the floor, rather than the first ray, using a simulated weight-bearing foot plate. Provisional fixation is then performed with a narrow-gauge K-wire (1.2–1.4 mm) once the desired position is achieved. A 2.7- to 3.5-mm lag screw is then placed in a distal/inferomedial to proximal/superolateral direction to achieve compression across the MTP joint. The provisional wire is removed before the screw is fully tightened to allow full compression. This construct is then neutralized with a precontoured dorsal plate, adhering to the principle of alignment, compression, and neutralization. At each stage the position of the hallux is checked and rechecked for the correct amount of valgus, dorsiflexion, and rotation; this position should be checked both clinically and fluoroscopically.

RESULTS

There are now several published series confirming the efficacy of this approach using a combination of dorsal plate, compression screw, and concentric cup-and-cone reamers. Kumar and colleagues[39] reported a fusion rate of 98% with a mean time to union of 3.1 months. Ellington and colleagues[40] reported an overall union rate of 87.9%, but this rose to 93.1% when the rheumatoid group was excluded. Goucher and Coughlin[41] also report good results, with satisfaction, union, and revision rates of 96%, 92%, and 4%, respectively.

IMPORTANT SURGICAL ISSUES

The spectrum of disease associated with a degenerate HV is wide, and recognition of this and variation of a standard technique is essential if a good outcome is to be achieved.

Poor Bone Quality

Osteoporosis remains a challenge when undertaking fusion procedures, not least in the first MTP joint where surface area is small, load is high, and leverage significant. The use of 2 screws, staples, or multiple wires can suffice in bone of reasonable quality, but this is not so in the case of osteoporosis. The authors avoid plaster casts and rigid splints following first MTP joint fusion, and this is achieved by modifying fixation when bone quality is poor.

Locking plates may provide an advantage in this situation, but are not infallible. Occasionally, if bone quality is very poor and fixation remains suspect, the authors have found that the addition of a 2-mm K-wire inserted in a retrograde fashion along the first ray, across the joints, increases stability and confidence in the construct.[6] This technique is a modification of that of Mann who used threaded Steinmann pins when he found bone stock to be inadequate. However, removal may prove to be difficult, and modification using a smooth wire to supplement plate fixation achieves a similar result in these unusual cases. Wire care needs to be meticulous, and removal at 4 weeks is often sufficient.

Severe Hallux Valgus Angle

In long-standing severe HV, the adductors of the proximal phalanx contract, especially in the severe rheumatoid forefoot. The hallux deformity is usually associated with dislocation and destruction of the lesser MTP joints, so significant shortening can be used in the first ray because similar shortening will occur in the lesser toes following excision arthroplasty procedures (Stainsby, Fowler, and so forth).[42–44] The authors' experience is that the most proximal corner of the valgus proximal phalanx is likely to be the level to which the first metatarsal will require shortening. This level maintains the continuity of the adductors and maximizes the correction of the IMA (**Figs. 3** and **4**).

If the surgery is to the first ray only then some length can be retained, but care should be taken to ensure that the blood supply to the toe remains satisfactory. If this still leaves the first ray significantly shorter than the lesser rays, the joint will need to be fused in less dorsiflexion to ensure that loading through the first ray is achieved.

Poorly Correcting Intermetatarsal Angle

The use of additional basal procedures is rarely indicated. Although Coughlin suggests an additional metatarsal osteotomy may rarely be necessary, he does not quantify this.[2] There are, however, some situations whereby an additional procedure may feasibly be required.

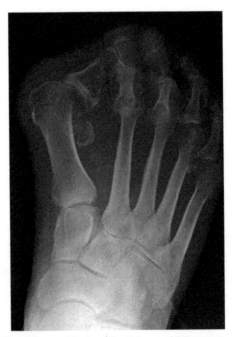

Fig. 3. Very severe hallux valgus with dorsally dislocated 2/3 metatarsophalangeal joints.

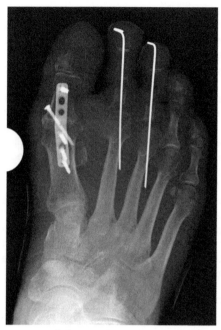

Fig. 4. Postoperative appearance following first metatarsophalangeal joint fusion and 2/3 toes Stainsby procedure.

1. As correction of the IMA relies on an intact adductor tendon, when using fusion to salvage failed HV surgery, one may find that the adductor has been divided.
2. If the basal joint is not mobile, for example, secondary to metatarsocuneiform arthrosis, correction of the hallux alone will lead to a broad forefoot, difficulty with shoe fit, and poor cosmesis, with a large gap between hallux and second toe.

To correct the IMA in these situations requires a metatarsal osteotomy, basal osteotomy, or Lapidus type fusion.

The authors have only identified one series that uses additional procedures routinely. Rippstein and colleagues[45] treated a cohort of patients, all of whom had a severe IMA of greater than 15°, undertaking preparation and temporary fixation of the first MTP joint. If the IMA remained greater than 10° an additional procedure was undertaken, either a Mau osteotomy or modified Lapidus fusion of the first tarsometatarsal joint. Although they showed good radiographic results with this approach (mean IMA correcting from 18.8° to 4.6° and HV angle from 49.9° to 9.7° postoperatively), the study had neither a control group nor randomization to prove or disprove the clinical necessity for the additional procedure.

In those patients with a severe deformity, it should be borne in mind that the IMA may not correct fully, although in most cases the correction will be adequate. However, but if it is considered intraoperatively that the correction is inadequate, an additional procedure may be undertaken.

Infected Bunion

The patient with an infected bunion needs to be fully assessed before attempting surgical intervention. This evaluation includes coexisting disease (diabetes, gout), perfusion (large and small vessel disease), neuropathy, and shoe wear. Conservative measures are often successful when infection is draining, there is sufficient perfusion to deliver adequate concentrations of antibiotics, and pressure is relieved. When osteomyelitis is present, especially in an immunocompromised host (eg, with diabetes), conservative eradication of the infection is difficult and surgery may be required.

Excision of the overlying ulcer, bursa, and bunion is required to debride the infected area. If the patient is low demand, poorly compliant, and incapable of protective weight bearing, this can be combined with excision of the proximal 50% of the proximal phalanx (Keller procedure).[46] Following a thorough washout, the surgical extensions are closed but the excised ulcer is left open. A pack can be inserted for 48 hours or a negative pressure-wound closure system applied. Appropriate antibiotics are used for 2 to 4 weeks, depending on the associated immune compromise and decrease in blood levels of inflammatory markers. The patient can fully weight bear in a bandage and stiff-soled sandal.

If the patient is higher demand, compliant, and capable of protective weight bearing, only the debridement is undertaken. Once closure has occurred, in 4 to 8 weeks, more definitive surgery can be undertaken such as a metatarsal osteotomy or first MTP joint fusion. Before this second stage of surgery, the wound should be clean and healed, and antibiotics discontinued. Microbiological guidance should be sought and biopsies sent at the time of surgery. Appropriate prophylactic antibiotics should be used.

Associated Interphalangeal Joint Arthritis

Fusion of both the first MTP joint and interphalangeal (IP) joint is technically difficult and poorly tolerated by the higher-demand patient. Toe pushoff is prevented and the nonunion rate is high. Mann and Oates describe a technique using a threaded Steinmann pin, and an extended locking plate can achieve the same aim, but patient satisfaction is poor.[8] The authors' preference is to maintain movement in at least one of the joints. In the lower-demand patient, this can be achieved using an IP joint fusion with a Keller procedure.[46] In the higher-demand patient, a judgment has to be made as to whether more conservative surgery to the first MTP joint would suffice. If so, an IP joint fusion can be undertaken together with a first MTP joint cheilectomy with a metatarsal osteotomy. If the subsequent correction is good but arthritic pain remains, joint replacement at a later date or conversion to a Keller procedure could be an option.

Smoking

There is good evidence that patients who smoke are at higher risk of wound problems and delayed union.[47,48] The preoperative cessation time is related to a reduced risk, but even stoppage on the day before surgery can have a significant effect. Before informed consent, smokers should be given cessation advice and the reasons why it is important. The authors do not deny surgery to smokers, but clear advice on the increased risks is given and surgery can be delayed while an attempt is made to stop smoking.

FUNCTIONAL OUTCOMES
Pedobarograph and Gait Changes

Fusion of the first MTP joint is usually successful, providing robust correction of the first ray, realigning flexor and extensor tendons, and increasing the contribution to pushoff.[49] The reduction in pain from the arthritic joint and reduced rubbing following bunion removal significantly contribute to improved function. When high function is required, including running and sprinting, fusion of the first MTP joint is the procedure of choice once HV has developed into advanced osteoarthritis.

However, the gait changes are not all positive, and DeFrino and colleagues[49] have shown that the inability to dorsiflex the joint leads to a reduced step length and reduced ankle plantarflexion at pushoff. In practice, reduction in pain and resultant improved function far outweighs these abnormalities found on gait analysis, but the effects should be considered when counseling athletes.

Shoewear considerations are important, especially if the patient wishes to wear a higher heel. Most can tolerate a heel up to 4 cm (1.5 inches), but more than this significantly loads the IP joint, leading to pain and reduced function. The authors do not advocate increasing the fusion dorsiflexion angle to facilitate higher heel usage, because this results in prominence and rubbing of the IP joint in flatter shoes and reduced or no pushoff from the terminal phalanx. The use of rocker profile soles, as found on some trainers and walking boots, improves rollover and may improve function with more normal ankle kinematics.

Time to Fusion

Time to solid fusion is variable, and factors such as surgical technique, patient compliance, and smoking will affect the outcome. However, Hyer and colleagues[50] assessed 4 plating techniques that were unable to show statistical difference but averaged 90% radiologic fusion at 8 weeks between the plates. The authors' preference is to assess the patient clinically and radiologically at 6 weeks and, if fusion is progressing well, to start weaning into more normal shoewear at this stage, avoiding running until 12 weeks and contact sports until 16 weeks. Appropriate shoewear can shorten these times if patient compliance is good.

Return to Work

Sedentary work can safely be undertaken once the wound has healed, from 2 weeks, although transport to and from work often delays this. Moderate activity at work can be commenced at 6 to 8 weeks, depending on shoewear, and resumption of heavy work may require 10 to 12 weeks.

Driving

Advice regarding driving should be provided with caution, as it is the responsibility of patients to ensure that they are able to control the vehicle safely at all times. However, the ability to perform an emergency stop without compromising reaction time following first metatarsal osteotomy was found to be 6 weeks.[51] The integrity of the fusion site of the first MTP joint would require reasonable bony union, which would be expected after 8 weeks.

SUMMARY

Fusion of the first MTP joint should be considered when managing either severe HV or more moderate HV associated with degenerative changes. It is also useful in patients for whom primary HV surgery has failed. Pitfalls include malposition and difficulty achieving and maintaining correction in those with poor bone quality or very severe deformities. Strategies to manage these situations are discussed herein.

REFERENCES

1. Perera AM, Mason L, Stephens MM. The pathogenesis of hallux valgus. J Bone Joint Surg Am 2011;93(17):1650–61. http://dx.doi.org/10.2106/JBJS.H.01630.
2. Coughlin MJ. Hallux valgus. J Bone Joint Surg Am 1996;78(6):932–66.

3. Shereff MJ. Pathophysiology, anatomy, and biomechanics of hallux valgus. Orthopedics 1990;13(9):939–45.

4. Scranton PE, Rutkowski R. Anatomic variations in the first ray: part I. Anatomic aspects related to bunion surgery. Clin Orthop 1980;151:244–55.

5. Robinson AH, Limbers JP. Modern concepts in the treatment of hallux valgus. J Bone Joint Surg Br 2005;87(8):1038–45. http://dx.doi.org/10.1302/0301-620X.87B8.16467.

6. Coughlin MJ, Grebing BR, Jones CP. Arthrodesis of the first metatarsophalangeal joint for idiopathic hallux valgus: intermediate results. Foot Ankle Int 2005;26(10):783–92.

7. Mann RA. Decision-making in bunion surgery. Instr Course Lect 1990;39:3–13.

8. Mann RA, Oates JC. Arthrodesis of the first metatarsophalangeal joint. Foot Ankle 1980;1(3):159–66.

9. Coughlin MJ. Rheumatoid forefoot reconstruction. A long-term follow-up study. J Bone Joint Surg Am 2000;82(3):322–41. PMID: 10724225.

10. Tourné Y, Saragaglia D, Zattara A, et al. Hallux valgus in the elderly: metatarsophalangeal arthrodesis of the first ray. Foot Ankle Int 1997;18(4):195–8.

11. Wu KK. First metatarsophalangeal fusion in the salvage of failed hallux abducto valgus operations. J Foot Ankle Surg 1994;33(4):383–95.

12. Desmarchelier R, Besse JL, Fessy MH. Scarf osteotomy versus metatarsophalangeal arthrodesis in forefoot first ray disorders: comparison of functional outcomes. Orthop Traumatol Surg Res 2012;98(Suppl 6):S77–84. http://dx.doi.org/10.1016/j.otsr.2012.04.016.

13. Bock P, Kristen KH, Kröner A, et al. Hallux valgus and cartilage degeneration in the first metatarsophalangeal joint. J Bone Joint Surg Br 2004;86(5):669–73.

14. Coughlin MJ. Arthrodesis of the first metatarsophalangeal joint with mini-fragment plate fixation. Orthopedics 1990;13(9):1037–44.

15. Harrison M, Harvey F. Arthrodesis of the first metatarsophalangeal joint for hallux valgus and rigidus. J Bone Joint Surg Am 1963;45:471–80.

16. Humbert JL, Bourbonnière C, Laurin CA. Metatarsophalangeal fusion for hallux valgus: indications and effect on the first metatarsal ray. Can Med Assoc J 1979; 120(8):937–41, 956.

17. Mckeever DC. Arthrodesis of the first metatarsophalangeal joint for hallux valgus, hallux rigidus, and metatarsus primus varus. J Bone Joint Surg Am 1952;34(1):129–34.

18. Moynihan FJ. Arthrodesis of the metatarso-phalangeal joint of the great toe. J Bone Joint Surg Br 1967;49(3):544–51.

19. Curtis MJ, Myerson M, Jinnah RH, et al. Arthrodesis of the first metatarsophalangeal joint: a biomechanical study of internal fixation techniques. Foot Ankle 1993;14(7):395–9.

20. Kelikian AS. Technical considerations in hallux metatarsal-phalangeal arthrodesis. Foot Ankle Clin 2005;10(1):167–90. http://dx.doi.org/10.1016/j.fcl.2004.11.002.

21. Choudhary RK, Theruvil B, Taylor GR. First metatarsophalangeal joint arthrodesis: a new technique of internal fixation by using memory compression staples. J Foot Ankle Surg 2004;43(5):312–7. http://dx.doi.org/10.1053/j.jfas.2004.07.003.

22. Besse J-L, Chouteau J, Laptoiu D. Arthrodesis of the first metatarsophalangeal joint with ball and cup reamers and osteosynthesis with pure titanium staples Radiological evaluation of a continuous series of 54 cases. Foot Ankle Surg 2010;16(1):32–7. http://dx.doi.org/10.1016/j.fas.2009.03.008.

23. Raymakers R, Waugh W. The treatment of metatarsalgia with hallux valgus. J Bone Joint Surg Br 1971;53(4):684–7.
24. Flavin R, Stephens MM. Arthrodesis of the first metatarsophalangeal joint using a dorsal titanium contoured plate. Foot Ankle Int 2004;25(11):783–7.
25. Mann RA, Katcherian DA. Relationship of metatarsophalangeal joint fusion on the intermetatarsal angle. Foot Ankle 1989;10(1):8–11.
26. Von Salis-Soglio G, Thomas W. Arthrodesis of the metatarsophalangeal joint of the great toe. Arch Orthop Trauma Surg 1979;95(1–2):7–12.
27. Brodsky JW, Passmore RN, Pollo FE, et al. Functional outcome of arthrodesis of the first metatarsophalangeal joint using parallel screw fixation. Foot Ankle Int 2005;26(2):140–6.
28. Buranosky DJ, Taylor DT, Sage RA, et al. First metatarsophalangeal joint arthrodesis: quantitative mechanical testing of six-hole dorsal plate versus crossed screw fixation in cadaveric specimens. J Foot Ankle Surg 2001;40(4):208–13.
29. Politi J, John H, Njus G, et al. First metatarsal-phalangeal joint arthrodesis: a biomechanical assessment of stability. Foot Ankle Int 2003;24(4):332–7. PMID: 12735376.
30. Bennett GL, Kay DB, Sabatta J. First metatarsophalangeal joint arthrodesis: an evaluation of hardware failure. Foot Ankle Int 2005;26(8):593–6.
31. Hunt KJ, Ellington JK, Anderson RB, et al. Locked versus nonlocked plate fixation for hallux MTP arthrodesis. Foot Ankle Int 2011;32(7):704–9.
32. Hunt KJ, Barr CR, Lindsey DP, et al. Locked versus nonlocked plate fixation for first metatarsophalangeal arthrodesis: a biomechanical investigation. Foot Ankle Int 2012;33(11):984–90. http://dx.doi.org/10.3113/FAI.2012.0984.
33. Bottlang M, Doornink J, Lujan TJ, et al. Effects of construct stiffness on healing of fractures stabilized with locking plates. J Bone Joint Surg Am 2010;92(Suppl 2): 12–22. http://dx.doi.org/10.2106/JBJS.J.00780.
34. Riggs SA Jr, Johnson EW Jr. McKeever arthrodesis for the painful hallux. Foot Ankle 1983;3(5):248–53.
35. Pydah SK, Toh EM, Sirikonda SP, et al. Intermetatarsal angular change following fusion of the first metatarsophalangeal joint. Foot Ankle Int 2009;30(5):415–8. http://dx.doi.org/10.3113/FAI.2009.0415.
36. Cronin JJ, Limbers JP, Kutty S, et al. Intermetatarsal angle after first metatarsophalangeal joint arthrodesis for hallux valgus. Foot Ankle Int 2006;27(2):104–9.
37. Sung W, Kluesner AJ, Irrgang J, et al. Radiographic outcomes following primary arthrodesis of the first metatarsophalangeal joint in hallux abductovalgus deformity. J Foot Ankle Surg 2010;49(5):446–51. http://dx.doi.org/10.1053/j.jfas.2010.06.007.
38. Dayton P, Lopiccolo J, Kiley J. Reduction of the intermetatarsal angle after first metatarsophalangeal joint arthrodesis in patients with moderate and severe metatarsus primus adductus. J Foot Ankle Surg 2002;41(5):316–9.
39. Kumar S, Pradhan R, Rosenfeld PF. First metatarsophalangeal arthrodesis using a dorsal plate and a compression screw. Foot Ankle Int 2010;31(9):797–801. http://dx.doi.org/10.3113/FAI.2010.0797.
40. Ellington JK, Jones CP, Cohen BE, et al. Review of 107 hallux MTP joint arthrodesis using dome-shaped reamers and a stainless-steel dorsal plate. Foot Ankle Int 2010;31(5):385–90. http://dx.doi.org/10.3113/FAI.2010.0385.
41. Goucher NR, Coughlin MJ. Hallux metatarsophalangeal joint arthrodesis using dome-shaped reamers and dorsal plate fixation: a prospective study. Foot Ankle Int 2006;27(11):869–76.
42. Briggs P, Stainsby G. Metatarsal head preservation in forefoot arthroplasty and the correction of severe claw toe deformity. Foot Ankle Surg 2001;7(2):93–101.

43. Stainsby G, Briggs P. Proceedings of the British Orthopaedic Association, Rhodes, May 2-6, 1989. Modified Keller's type procedure for the lateral four toes. J Bone Joint Surg Br 1990;72:529–33.

44. Fowler AW. A method of forefoot reconstruction. J Bone Joint Surg Br 1959;41:507–13.

45. Rippstein PF, Park YU, Naal FD. Combination of first metatarsophalangeal joint arthrodesis and proximal correction for severe hallux valgus deformity. Foot Ankle Int 2012;33(5):400–5. http://dx.doi.org/10.3113/FAI.2012.0400.

46. Keller W. The surgical treatment of bunions and hallux valgus. New York Med J 1904;80:741–2.

47. Cobb TK, Gabrielsen TA, Campbell DC, et al. Cigarette smoking and nonunion after ankle arthrodesis. Foot Ankle Int 1994;15(2):64–7. PMID: 7981802.

48. Krannitz KW, Fong HW, Fallat LM, et al. The effect of cigarette smoking on radiographic bone healing after elective foot surgery. J Foot Ankle Surg 2009;48(5):525–7. http://dx.doi.org/10.1053/j.jfas.2009.04.008.

49. DeFrino PF, Brodsky JW, Pollo FE, et al. First metatarsophalangeal arthrodesis: a clinical, pedobarographic and gait analysis study. Foot Ankle Int 2002;23(6):496–502.

50. Hyer CF, Scott RT, Swiatek M. A retrospective comparison of four plate constructs for first metatarsophalangeal joint fusion: static plate, static plate with lag screw, locked plate, and locked plate with lag screw. J Foot Ankle Surg 2012;51(3):285–7. http://dx.doi.org/10.1053/j.jfas.2012.02.006.

51. Holt G, Kay M, McGrory R, et al. Emergency brake response time after first metatarsal osteotomy. J Bone Joint Surg Am 2008;90(8):1660–4. http://dx.doi.org/10.2106/JBJS.G.00552.

Recurrence of Hallux Valgus
A Review

Steven M. Raikin, MD[a],*, Adam G. Miller, MD[b], Joseph Daniel, DO[a]

KEYWORDS

- Hallux valgus • Recurrence • Revision • Bunion

KEY POINTS

- Pain in the setting of recurrent deformity is the primary indication for revision hallux valgus surgery.
- Surgery for recurrence relies on the ability of the surgeon to determine the cause of the recurrence.
- Although the relevance of tarsometatarsal hypermobility has been challenged in the development and management of primary hallux valgus deformity, once a recurrence develops, closer attention is advised in assessing this joint.
- Revision surgery for recurrence should use a technique at least as powerful as that of the primary intervention.

EPIDEMIOLOGY

Complications following hallux valgus (HV) surgery have been reported to be as high as 50%,[1,2] with one of the most common complications being recurrent HV.[3] However, rates of HV recurrence vary in the literature from 2.7% to 16%.[3-7] Lagaay and colleagues[8] reviewed revision rates for recurrent HV in a multicenter study following primary chevron osteotomies (1.85%) versus Lapidus procedures (2.92%) and closing base wedge osteotomy (2.94%), finding no statistical difference in revision rates over various methods of primary HV correction. No description was given for the severity of the deformity before the index procedure or why that particular index procedure was chosen.

The cause of recurrent HV is usually multifactorial, and includes patient-related factors such as preoperative anatomic predisposition, medical comorbidities, and compliance with postcorrection instructions, as well as surgical factors such as the choice of the appropriate procedure to address the given HV pattern and the technical competency of performing the corrective procedure (**Table 1**).

[a] Rothman Institute, 925 Chestnut Street, Philadelphia, PA 19107, USA; [b] Beacon Orthopaedics and Sports Medicine, 500 East Business Way, Cincinnati, OH 45241, USA
* Corresponding author.
E-mail address: steven.raikin@rothmaninstitute.com

Foot Ankle Clin N Am 19 (2014) 259–274
http://dx.doi.org/10.1016/j.fcl.2014.02.008
foot.theclinics.com

Table 1 Risk factors for recurrence	
Anatomic	Skeletal immaturity
	Hypermobility
	Congruent joint (high DMAA)
Nonanatomic (systemic)	Hyperlaxity (Ehlers-Danlos, Marfan)
	Rheumatoid arthritis
	Hypothyroidism
	Gout
	Neuromuscular condition
	Cerebrovascular accident
Social	Smoking
	Noncompliance
	Continued high-heel shoewear
Surgical	Wrong surgery
	Undercorrection
	Technical

Abbreviation: DMAA, distal metatarsal articular angle.

Patient Risk Factors: Anatomic

There is a paucity of literature examining patients' risk factors related to the recurrence of HV deformity following correction. Like primary HV, recurrent HV can occur in the setting of a family history of HV. Surgical correction in skeletally immature (adolescent- or juvenile-onset HV) patients have historically been associated with a high recurrence rate of up to 50%.[9] Coughlin and Roger,[10] however, challenged this notion, demonstrating a 10% recurrence rate (6 of 60 feet) after an average of 5 years' follow-up, concluding that the appropriately performed and selected procedures can result in successful outcomes with low recurrence rates in this population group.

In addition, younger patients tend to have a high degree of concomitant metatarsus adductus. Although this finding is not a predictor of recurrence, it does make correction technically more difficult, predisposing to inadequate deformity correction, which can lead to higher recurrence rates (**Fig. 1**). Similarly, a high distal metatarsal articular angle (DMAA) is frequently seen in juvenile-onset and adolescent-onset HV patients. To maintain a congruent joint while adequately correcting the HV angular deformity is most successfully achieved through a double osteotomy (2 separate levels and planes of deformity correction) to avoid recurrence or a noncongruent joint leading to arthritis. These findings may also be present in adult HV patients, and similar care in addressing these factors should be used in treating these deformities.

Hypermobility of the first tarsometatarsal (TMT) joint remains controversial regarding its existence and relevance in patients with HV. If the joint is hypermobile, particularly in the coronal plane, a higher recurrence rate may result (**Fig. 2**).[11]

Nonanatomic Patient Factors

In addition to bone and joint morphologic features that may predispose to recurrence of an HV deformity following surgical correction, factors affecting the supporting structures of the first metatarsophalangeal (MTP) joint can also lead to recurrence. Generalized hyperlaxity conditions, such as Ehlers-Danlos syndrome or Marfan syndrome, result in laxity at the first MTP and TMT joints, which will predispose the patient to recurrence of deformity and an unsuccessful long-term outcome.

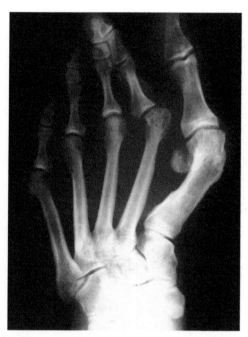

Fig. 1. Recurrence of hallux valgus (HV) with malunion of a distal metatarsal osteotomy in a patient with metatarsus adductus.

Medical conditions implicated in recurrent HV include rheumatoid arthritis (RA), hypothyroidism, seronegative arthropathies, and gout,[12] caused by loss of synovial capsular support as a result of inflammatory arthritis or invasive crystalline conditions such as gout. Neuromuscular conditions, especially when resulting in muscular spasticity that is not overcome during the primary procedure, can contribute to recurrence. These disorders include juvenile conditions such as cerebral palsy, Down syndrome and muscular dystrophies, hereditary neuropathies (such as Charcot-Marie-Tooth/ hereditary motor sensory neuropathy), and adult-onset conditions as seen following polio or cerebrovascular accidents.[12] Arthrodesis procedures used to correct HV reveal a much lower recurrence rate in such patient populations.

Patient-driven social risk factors should be noted and discussed with the patient, as these are generally controllable by the patient. Smoking has been associated with nonunion in Lapidus procedures and with minor wound complications following revision surgery.[13] Postoperative patient compliance has been significantly associated with failure of other lower extremity surgery.[14,15] To the authors' knowledge, this has only been noted anecdotally in reference to HV.[16]

Early forefoot weight bearing and lack of dressing maintenance are both potential pitfalls in the postoperative management of a primary HV correction. In addition, in the same manner that certain shoes (high heels; narrow toe box) predispose to the development of primary HV, continued wear following correction may also contribute to recurrence.[12]

Surgeon-Related and Surgery-Related Risk Factors

There are more than 100 different described procedures to address HV deformities. The selection of which procedure should be used for any given patient needs to be carefully made by diligent assessment of the preoperative findings. The adage that

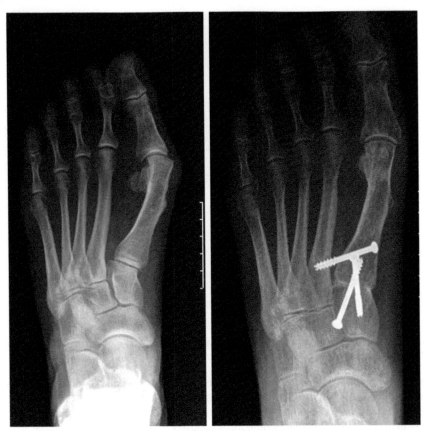

Fig. 2. Recurrent HV after distal osteotomy with hypermobility at the tarsometatarsal joint proximally. (*Left*) The joint has subluxed laterally with weight bearing. (*Right*) Correction with fusion.

the procedure should fit the deformity, rather than the deformity being made to fit the procedure, remains ever true in HV correction.

Recent weight-bearing images of the foot are of critical importance in preoperative planning. A study conducted by Okuda and colleagues[4] looked at the relationship between the HV angle (HVA) and the intermetatarsal angle (IMA), and showed that a preoperative HVA greater than 40° correlated with a more likely recurrence rate, whereas an immediate postoperative HVA of less than 15° and an IMA of less than 10° was associated with a lower likelihood of revision surgery.

Sesamoid position has also been implicated as a risk factor for recurrence of HV.[17] The Hardy and Clapham grading scheme examines lateral displacement of the medial sesamoid, and is strongly associated with recurrence. This study reinforces the need for adequate soft-tissue release during the Modified McBride portion of HV surgery to ensure appropriate sesamoid position.

REASONS FOR RECURRENCE
Presenting Symptoms

Pain in the setting of recurrent deformity is the primary indication for revision HV surgery.[18] Proper identification of the location of pain is important. Medially based pain can be a consequence of inadequate resection of the eminence, whereas plantar pain may be due to sesamoiditis, sesamoid arthritis, or malreduction of the sesamoids at the index procedure. If deformity recurs but is not painful, one should apply similar reasoning to that when evaluating a primary deformity, and surgery should not be performed.

Choice of Surgery

The inappropriate choice of a procedure at the time of the index operation is a relatively common cause for recurrence, pain, and the need to consider revision surgery. Accurate preoperative measurement of the deformity using weight-bearing images and understanding the power and limitations of each surgical option will likely lead to selection of the most appropriate procedure.[19]

It is not the purpose of this review to discuss in detail the algorithm for appropriate selection of the primary procedure, which is discussed elsewhere in this issue. However, it is important to state that an underpowered procedure that cannot achieve or maintain an appropriate correction will lead to a much higher recurrence rate. A Silver (simple) bunionectomy whereby the medial eminence is shaved down but neither the contracted lateral structures are rebalanced nor the intermetatarsal angle corrected will fail to obtain long-term correction of the HV deformity despite an appropriate medial capsulorrhaphy **(Fig. 3)**.[20]

Austin and Leventen[21] reviewed 300 distal chevron osteotomies and found a 10% recurrence rate of HV when the deformity was considered mild to moderate. Johnson and colleagues[19] cautioned against using a chevron osteotomy with an IMA greater than 25°. The Keller-Brandes resection arthroplasty of the first metatarsal has historically shown poor results, with late recurrence and instability.[22] This procedure should be considered with caution and used only in the low-demand patient. Late recurrence should be addressed with a first metatarsophalangeal joint arthrodesis.

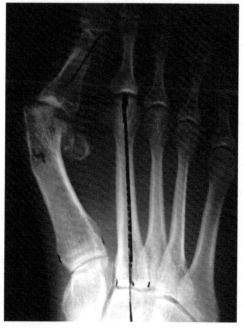

Fig. 3. Failed Silver-type procedure with recurrent deformity.

Surgical Technique

In addition to selecting the appropriate procedure for the particular HV deformity, technical competence in performing the procedure is essential in avoiding recurrence and failure. From an osseous standpoint, the lack of adequate lateral displacement of the metatarsal head during a chevron procedure, as well as osteotomy malunion, nonunion, or osteotomy fracture, may occur. An inadequate resection of the medial eminence or a too aggressive resection can also be problematic.

In the presence of an abnormal IMA, primary correction of the HV deformity should be obtained through bony realignment. Although one should not rely on the capsulorrhaphy alone for correction, incomplete release of soft tissue from the dorsal first web space or improper medial capsular plication can lead to recurrence or a hallux varus deformity. Even with powerful proximal metatarsal osteotomies, inadequate correction of the intermetatarsal angle will result in recurrence. In a long-term follow-up study (mean 5.5 years) of successful HV corrections with more than 85% satisfaction, a crescentic proximal metatarsal (MT) osteotomy with distal soft-tissue release was shown to lose 3.8° of HV angle correction and 1.4° of IMA correction.[23]

One must then consider the degree of correction at the time of primary HV surgery, acknowledging that some relapse may occur. The prescribed technique must be adequately strong in preventing undercorrection. Lastly, poor implant selection or poor use of the implant may be a factor.

Postoperative Complications

Avascular necrosis of the MT head following a distal osteotomy has been reported.[24] This necrosis can occur when performing a distal soft-tissue procedure in conjunction with a Chevron osteotomy. An aggressive plantar cut may also disrupt soft tissue plantarly, disrupting blood supply of digital arteries.

Nonunion can occur following MTP fusion or Lapidus procedures, with rates from 2% to 13% being reported.[25,26] Less commonly, nonunion can follow MT osteotomies. Rates of nonunion in MTP fusion were reported at 86.9% in one study, with only 3 of 14 patients going on to require another procedure.[26] Again, symptoms should be assessed when diagnosing nonunion and determining subsequent treatment. An asymptomatic pseudarthrosis at the first MTP joint may not require further treatment.

PRIMARY HV ALGORITHM

Primary HV surgical treatment can be best elucidated by following clinical and radiographic indications, summarized in **Fig. 4**.

TREATMENT OF REVISION HALLUX VALGUS

The evaluation of the patient with a recurrent HV deformity entails determining the location of pain, what generates pain and the degree of the deformity, similar to managing a primary HV deformity. The difference is to ascertain why the deformity recurred. One has to try to ascertain whether the initial surgery was poorly planned or performed, or whether patient factors were largely contributory. For instance, was the patient noncompliant, was the true extent of the deformity missed and thus the surgery performed inadequate (**Fig. 5**), or was there some underlying medical condition missed or has a new condition occurred? Similarly to a primary HV, deformity in the absence of pain should be treated in a nonoperative fashion.

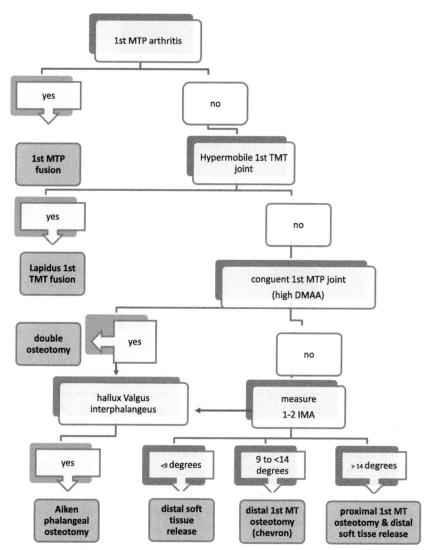

Fig. 4. Algorithm for primary and revision HV deformity correction. DMAA, distal metatarsal articular angle; IMA, intermetatarsal angle; MT, metatarsal; MTP, metatarsophalangeal; TMT, tarsometatarsal.

Nonoperative Treatment

Consistent with primary treatment of HV deformity, first-line treatment should involve a discussion of a nonoperative course.[6] The primary motivation must be discerned to satisfy and adequately treat the patient. If pain with ambulation is not a primary concern, revision HV surgery is most likely not indicated.[27] Other treatment modalities and causes of pain should be entertained.

Operative Treatment

As already mentioned, the revision surgical procedure for management of a symptomatic recurrent HV should be chosen according to the same evaluator criteria in

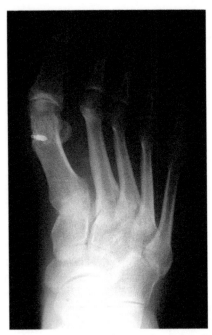

Fig. 5. Distal HV correction with inadequate chevron for deformity.

selecting correction of a primary HV deformity. These surgeries include MTP fusion for arthritic and unstable MTP joints; first tarsometatarsal fusion (Lapidus procedure) if this joint is hypermobile and this is thought to have resulted in the recurrence of the deformity; or first metatarsal osteotomies to correct recurrent or undercorrected inter-metatarsal angular deformities.

Additional procedures that may be considered include medial closing wedge hallux proximal phalangeal osteotomy (Aiken procedure) for uncorrected HV interphalan-geus; and double osteotomies to correct malunions or uncorrected high DMAA defor-mities with congruent MTP joints.

In addition, one must always consider the secondary or associated involvement of the lesser MTs and MTP joints that may occur as a result of the recurrent HV deformity, or secondary to an overshortened first MT from the primary procedure. This short-ening can also result during the revision procedure, and this must be taken into ac-count during the surgical planning.

Metatarsophalangeal Fusion

First-ray MTP fusion can be used in a variety of pathologic conditions as a salvage pro-cedure including RA, failed implants, neuromuscular disorders, hallux varus, and recurrent HV.[28] In addition, as previously mentioned, a recurrent HV after Keller (**Fig. 6**) resection is best managed surgically with an MTP fusion of the first ray.

This procedure was first described with success in 16 feet by Coughlin and Mann.[29] Vienne and colleagues[22] evaluated a series of these feet[29] with 2-year follow-up. Mean American Orthopaedic Foot and Ankle Society (AOFAS) scores significantly improved (from 44 to 85) and 72% of patients were pain free. There were 2 reported patients with pseudarthrosis on follow-up. Similar results were found by Machacek and col-leagues,[30] with 26 of 29 feet achieving fusion for Keller revision. In addition, a repeat Keller procedure has also shown to be tolerated poorly in midterm follow-up.[30]

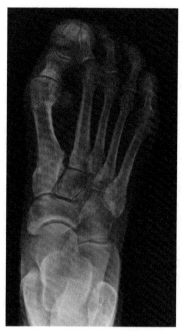

Fig. 6. Failed Keller resection with recurrence.

Another review expanded on the indications of MTP fusion in a revision setting, looking at 33 feet at an average follow-up of 8 years (range 1–22 years).[31] Four non-unions occurred, of which only 1 was symptomatic. With this long follow-up, 72% of patients rated their outcomes as good or excellent. The investigators concluded that although MTP fusion is a versatile procedure in treating nearly all types of recurrent HV deformities, the outcomes following revision surgery need to be tempered.

In addition, MTP fusion is not indicated in the patient with tarsometatarsal hypermobility, but is indicated for recurrent HV secondary to generalized hypermobility disorders such as Ehler-Danlos syndrome, and for patients with recurrent HV secondary to neuromuscular imbalance. It should obviously be considered the operation of choice if there is recurrence, without significant metatarsal osseous deformity, with secondary degenerative changes.

Lapidus Procedure

Fusion of the first TMT joint with correction of the intermetatarsal angle for correction of HV deformity was allegedly first described by Albrecht in 1911, but it was popularized by Lapidus in 1934.[32] In the revision situation the Lapidus procedure[33] can be used to address a previously undetected hypermobility of the first ray at the TMT joint.

The clinical examination should evaluate instability in both the sagittal and transverse planes. Plain radiographs may reveal incongruence of the first metatarsal–medial cuneiform (1 MTC) articulation with associated dorsal or medial bossing of the joint, or plantar divergence of the 1 MTC joint. Ellington reported on 25 feet undergoing Lapidus for revision[34] and reported that 96% of patients had signs of clinical hypermobility while 52% had radiographic signs of instability. At a minimum 1-year follow-up, 87% of patients reported good to excellent results.

In a revision setting, strength of potential correction using a Lapidus fusion is appealing. This technique applies to undercorrected HV surgery and initial poor selection of the initial procedure, as previously described. Coetzee and colleagues[11] described 26 patients with recurrent HV undergoing modified Lapidus with a variety of primary failed surgeries, only excluding Keller and Mayo primary resection surgeries.[13] This report consisted of patients with and without instability, demonstrating why the investigators referred to the Lapidus as "the final answer" in select patients. In this group, 5 of the patients did not demonstrate instability at the tarsometatarsal (TMT) joint. Regardless, 81% of patients were satisfied at final follow-up. Three patients with smoking history required revision for nonunion of the TMT joint.

Concerns with Lapidus include the learning curve in the revision setting, shortening of the first ray, high fusion nonunion rate, and longer recovery period. Once cartilage surfaces are denuded from the TMT joint, shortening of the first ray may create iatrogenic transfer metatarsalgia. Although this is apparent in primary settings, an emphasis must be placed on this complication in the revision setting because of the potential for an already shortened first ray from previous surgery.

Evaluating lesser MT at the time of revision surgery is indicated, and adding distal oblique shortening osteotomies of the lesser MT for first MT shortening of greater than 1 cm has been recommended. Greater than 2 cm of first MT shortening may require a bone-block interposition lengthening of the first MT.[13] The groups of Coetzee and Ellington[13,34] report shortening of 2.7 and 2.9 mm, respectively. One must also take care to position the TMT fusion in the appropriate degree of plantarflexion so as to create a balanced and plantigrade foot following surgery, thereby compensating for the aforementioned shortening.

First Metatarsal Osteotomy

MT osteotomy for revision HV surgery has been reported in the form of a proximal osteotomy or double osteotomy. Isolated distal MT osteotomy for revision surgery has not been reported, most likely because of strength of correction, blood supply to the MT head, and mechanism of failure.

Proximal osteotomy can be performed in a variety of methods including, but not limited to, Ludloff, crescentic, Scarf (**Fig. 7**), or opening wedge osteotomies (**Fig. 8**). Kitaoka and Patzer[16] reported on 14 feet undergoing revision with crescentic osteotomies for recurrent HV. Patients had previously undergone a chevron osteotomy or exostectomy with soft-tissue release. Complications included transfer metatarsalgia in 3 patients, recurrence in 1, and hallux varus in another. Overall, 3 patients considered their revision to have a poor outcome. Two of these patients had a dorsiflexed malunion at the osteotomy site, resulting from excessive shortening of the first MT.

The use of the Scarf procedure in the primary setting has been primarily for metatarsus primus varus, and the authors use this same algorithm for its use in revision surgery, excluding previous resection arthroplasties or cases of instability.[18] In this study, 39 feet underwent Scarf osteotomy for what the investigators concluded was recurrent HV resulting from failure to perform an osteotomy at the time of initial surgery. At a mean follow-up of 42 months, AOFAS scores improved significantly from a mean of 56 to 90 points, but 5 patients did have symptomatic hardware. One patient developed hallux varus while another had a second recurrence HV postoperatively.

A double osteotomy in the form of a distal short Scarf and proximal open wedge osteotomy has been reported in revision of an underpowered chevron procedure.[35] Ensuring there is no instability present and that the chosen osteotomy is strong enough to correct the metatarsus primus varus is paramount. For this reason, Sammarco and Idusuyi[12] have recommended only proximal osteotomies in a revision setting instead of a distal osteotomy surgery alone. In addition, there is no literature comparing various proximal osteotomies in a revision setting.

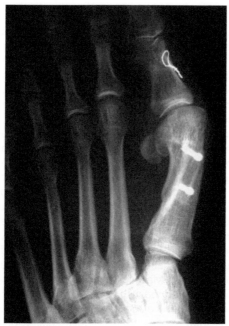

Fig. 7. Recurrent HV following correction using a Scarf osteotomy of the first metatarsal.

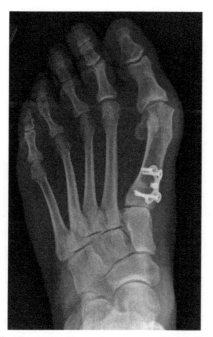

Fig. 8. Recurrent HV following correction using an opening wedge osteotomy of the first metatarsal.

DISCUSSION

When encountering a patient with complaints after HV surgery, one must first understand the primary reason for the visit. If pain is the primary complaint, this leads to the investigative process for determining why, despite a surgical attempt, this patient continues to experience symptoms. Only once the cause of the recurrence is identified may one effectively treat the underlying condition and symptoms. Just as the surgical technique for revision surgery is more technically challenging, so this process can require more expertise.

In assessing the underlying cause, the authors reference the same algorithm initially used during the primary procedure (see **Fig. 3**), with emphasis on assessment of previously undetected hypermobility of the first ray at the TMT joint clinically or radiographically. Although the relevance of TMT hypermobility has been challenged in the development and management of primary HV deformity,[36] once a recurrence develops, closer attention is advised in assessing this joint. Caveats to this algorithm include assessment of a painful first MT after Keller or Mayo resection. With either resection of the proximal phalanx (Keller) or metatarsal head (Mayo), the painful instability that may occur can only be salvaged with an MTP fusion of the first ray.

Other caveats include complications from the previous surgery that result in the eventual recurrence of deformity. Malunion of a fusion (see **Fig. 1**) or proximal osteotomy may result in a plantarflexed toe with which the patient may not be able to clear the floor during the swing phase of gait. More often the malunion is dorsiflexed, thereby decreasing the load applied to the medial column during weight bearing; this may result in transfer metatarsalgia, as previously mentioned.

Nonunion of a fusion can result in a stable pseudarthrosis or a painful first ray. In cases of painful nonunions, surgery is indicated for achieving fusion (**Fig. 9**). In patients with risk factors such as smoking or otherwise, bone graft or similar substitute may be warranted.

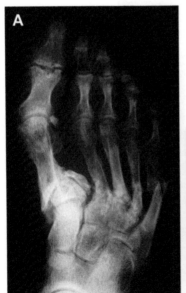
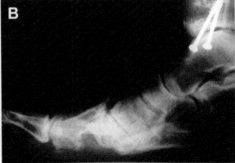

Fig. 9. (*A*) Anteroposterior and (*B*) lateral radiographs of a metatarsal nonunion following HV correction in a patient with rheumatoid arthritis.

Other complications that may not be obvious on clinical visit need to be considered, including initial postoperative compliance or continued inappropriate shoewear. If the initial surgery was appropriate and performed correctly, this should be a concern moving forward when planning a revision case, especially when considering a fusion-type procedure with longer time to healing.

Assuming that complications are not the cause of recurrence, one then can assess the deformity clinically and radiographically according to the aforementioned algorithm. Similarly to Sammarco and Idusuyi,[12] the authors would not recommend performing a less powerful operation than the primary HV surgery attempted. Failure constitutes the need for a surgery performed better, or a more powerful surgery. This point relates to 1 of the 2 major reasons for recurrence: underpowered surgery. In underpowered surgery the initial surgery did not technically achieve an appropriate outcome, or the correction was inadequate. These patients may undergo an operation similar to the primary one if tissue allows. For example, an underpowered proximal osteotomy might be revised with another proximal osteotomy. Otherwise, the patient may need to undergo a more powerful operation. In the example just mentioned, this would be a first MTP fusion or Lapidus procedure.

Wrong surgery is the other major reason for revision. When a patient undergoes a primary HV procedure that simply does not have the corrective capacity for the patient's deformity, one may say a more powerful surgery should have initially been performed (**Fig. 10**). Common examples of wrong surgery include a simple exostectomy with or without a Modified McBride distal soft-tissue release, or a distal chevron osteotomy for an intermetatarsal angle between the first and second MT of greater than 14°. These revisions can often be adequately treated with a more powerful intervention.

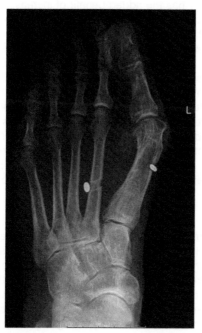

Fig. 10. Failure of a HV correction after suture bridge technique. In this patient, the initial deformity was too severe (intermetatarsal angle >14°).

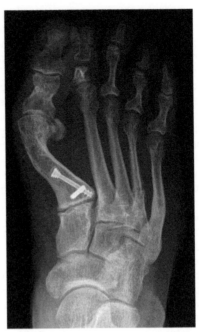

Fig. 11. Double osteotomy of the first metatarsal with malunion distally and inadequate correction proximally for a congruent HV deformity. Both aspects of this surgery were performed incorrectly.

Although larger surgery has the added benefit of increased correction potential, it maintains a longer postoperative course and the potential for increased complications. Therefore, the authors advocate the aforementioned thought process in determining which revision surgery is appropriate for a patient, applied on an individual basis. Patients need to be informed that outcomes of revision surgery, all be they good, are neither as positive nor as reliable as an appropriate primary corrective procedure could have been, and, as such, their expectations for their outcomes need to be realistic. Finally, the follow-up duration of most of the outcome studies on the management of primary or recurrent HV most commonly averages less than 5 years. Very little has been published about the time to develop a recurrence of an HV deformity following primary correction. In the study by Ellington and colleagues[34] on conversion to a Lapidus procedure, however, the time between the index procedure and the revision for recurrent HV deformity averaged 91 months (over a period of 7.5 years).

SUMMARY

Recurrence of HV deformity can be a common complication after corrective surgery. The cause of recurrent HV is usually multifactorial, and includes patient-related factors such as preoperative anatomic predispositions, medical comorbidities, compliance with postcorrection instructions, and surgical factors such as the choice of the appropriate procedure and technical competence (**Fig. 11**). For a successful outcome, this cause must be ascertained preoperatively. Revision surgery is technically more challenging, and potential complications and prolonged postoperative care should be discussed with the patient. Although the literature suggests a trend toward more fusion surgery (metatarsophalangeal fusion and Lapidus), this is not absolute. When choosing a corrective technique, revision surgery for recurrence should use a technique at least as powerful as that of the primary intervention.

REFERENCES

1. Thompson FM. Complications of hallux valgus surgery and salvage. Orthopedics 1990;13(9):1059–67.
2. Easley ME, Trnka HJ. Current concepts review: hallux valgus part II: operative treatment. Foot Ankle Int 2007;28(6):748–58.
3. Kilmartin TE, O'Kane C. Combined rotation scarf and Akin osteotomies for hallux valgus: a patient focussed 9 year follow up of 50 patients. J Foot Ankle Res 2010;3:2.
4. Okuda R, Kinoshita M, Yasuda T, et al. Hallux valgus angle as a predictor of recurrence following proximal metatarsal osteotomy. J Orthop Sci 2011;16(6): 760–4.
5. Lehman DE. Salvage of complications of hallux valgus surgery. Foot Ankle Clin 2003;8(1):15–35.
6. Coughlin MJ. Hallux valgus. J Bone Joint Surg Am 1996;78(6):932–66.
7. Robinson AH, Limbers JP. Modern concepts in the treatment of hallux valgus. J Bone Joint Surg Br 2005;87(8):1038–45.
8. Lagaay PM, Hamilton GA, Ford LA, et al. Rates of revision surgery using Chevron-Austin osteotomy, Lapidus arthrodesis, and closing base wedge osteotomy for correction of hallux valgus deformity. J Foot Ankle Surg 2008; 47(4):267–72.
9. Ball J, Sullivan JA. Treatment of the juvenile bunion by Mitchell osteotomy. Orthopedics 1985;8(10):1249–52.
10. Coughlin MJ. Roger A. Mann Award. Juvenile hallux valgus: etiology and treatment. Foot Ankle Int 1995;16(11):682–97.
11. Coetzee JC, Resig SG, Kuskowski M, et al. The Lapidus procedure as salvage after failed surgical treatment of hallux valgus. Surgical technique. J Bone Joint Surg Am 2004;86A(Suppl 1):30–6.
12. Sammarco GJ, Idusuyi OB. Complications after surgery of the hallux. Clin Orthop Relat Res 2001;(391):59–71.
13. Coetzee JC, Resig SG, Kuskowski M, et al. The Lapidus procedure as salvage after failed surgical treatment of hallux valgus: a prospective cohort study. J Bone Joint Surg Am 2003;85A(1):60–5.
14. Miller AG, Margules A, Raikin SM. Risk factors for wound complications after ankle fracture surgery. J Bone Joint Surg Am 2012;94(22):2047–52.
15. Osterhoff G, Boni T, Berli M. Recurrence of acute Charcot neuropathic osteoarthropathy after conservative treatment. Foot Ankle Int 2013;34(3):359–64.
16. Kitaoka HB, Patzer GL. Salvage treatment of failed hallux valgus operations with proximal first metatarsal osteotomy and distal soft-tissue reconstruction. Foot Ankle Int 1998;19(3):127–31.
17. Okuda R, Kinoshita M, Yasuda T, et al. Postoperative incomplete reduction of the sesamoids as a risk factor for recurrence of hallux valgus. J Bone Joint Surg Am 2009;91(7):1637–45.
18. Bock P, Lanz U, Kroner A, et al. The Scarf osteotomy: a salvage procedure for recurrent hallux valgus in selected cases. Clin Orthop Relat Res 2010;468(8): 2177–87.
19. Johnson KA, Cofield RH, Morrey BF. Chevron osteotomy for hallux valgus. Clin Orthop Relat Res 1979;(142):44–7.

20. Kitaoka HB, Franco MG, Weaver AL, et al. Simple bunionectomy with medial capsulorrhaphy. Foot Ankle 1991;12(2):86–91.

21. Austin DW, Leventen EO. A new osteotomy for hallux valgus: a horizontally directed "V" displacement osteotomy of the metatarsal head for hallux valgus and primus varus. Clin Orthop Relat Res 1981;(157):25–30.

22. Vienne P, Sukthankar A, Favre P, et al. Metatarsophalangeal joint arthrodesis after failed Keller-Brandes procedure. Foot Ankle Int 2006;27(11):894–901.

23. Dreeben S, Mann RA. Advanced hallux valgus deformity: long-term results utilizing the distal soft tissue procedure and proximal metatarsal osteotomy. Foot Ankle Int 1996;17(3):142–4.

24. Edwards WH. Avascular necrosis of the first metatarsal head. Foot Ankle Clin 2005;10(1):117–27.

25. Cottom JM, Vora AM. Fixation of lapidus arthrodesis with a plantar interfragmentary screw and medial locking plate: a report of 88 cases. J Foot Ankle Surg 2013; 52(4):465–9.

26. Bennett GL, Kay DB, Sabatta J. First metatarsophalangeal joint arthrodesis: an evaluation of hardware failure. Foot Ankle Int 2005;26(8):593–6.

27. Duan X, Kadakia AR. Salvage of recurrence after failed surgical treatment of hallux valgus. Arch Orthop Trauma Surg 2012;132(4):477–85.

28. Trnka HJ. Arthrodesis procedures for salvage of the hallux metatarsophalangeal joint. Foot Ankle Clin 2000;5(3):673–86, ix.

29. Coughlin MJ, Mann RA. Arthrodesis of the first metatarsophalangeal joint as salvage for the failed Keller procedure. J Bone Joint Surg Am 1987;69(1):68–75.

30. Machacek F Jr, Easley ME, Gruber F, et al. Salvage of the failed Keller resection arthroplasty. Surgical technique. J Bone Joint Surg Am 2005;87(Suppl 1(Pt 1)): 86–94.

31. Grimes JS, Coughlin MJ. First metatarsophalangeal joint arthrodesis as a treatment for failed hallux valgus surgery. Foot Ankle Int 2006;27(11):887–93.

32. Lapidus PW. The operative correction of the metatarsus primus varus in hallux valgus. Surg Gynecol Obstet 1934;58:183–91.

33. Lapidus PW. A quarter of a century of experience with the operative correction of the metatarsus varus primus in hallux valgus. Bull Hosp Joint Dis 1956;17(2): 404–21.

34. Ellington JK, Myerson MS, Coetzee JC, et al. The use of the Lapidus procedure for recurrent hallux valgus. Foot Ankle Int 2011;32(7):674–80.

35. Lim JB, Huntley JS. Revisional surgery for hallux valgus with serial osteotomies at two levels. ScientificWorldJournal 2011;11:657–61.

36. Coughlin MJ, Jones CP. Hallux valgus and first ray mobility. A prospective study. J Bone Joint Surg Am 2007;89(9):1887–98.

The Treatment of Iatrogenic Hallux Varus

Mark B. Davies, BM, FRCS(Orth)*, Chris M. Blundell, MD, FRCS(Orth)

KEYWORDS

• Hallux varus • Iatrogenic • Tenodesis • Corrective osteotomy

KEY POINTS

• Though uncommon, iatrogenic hallux varus is most often the result of overresection of the medial eminence, overtranslation of an osteotomy, overrelease of the lateral soft tissues, or overtightening of the medial tissues.
• Iatrogenic hallux varus is not always symptomatic, as the degree of deformity can be well tolerated.
• For soft-tissue reconstructions, releases have little role to play unless minor deformity is detected early on and the longevity of tendon transfer and tenodesis remains unknown.
• For bony reconstruction, arthrodesis is the recommended salvage technique.

INTRODUCTION

Hallux varus is a deformity characterized by medial deviation of the great toe secondary to an imbalance of the musculotendinous units that cross the first metatarsophalangeal joint (MTPJ). Though rare, hallux varus can present in adolescence as a result of an underlying neuromuscular imbalance such as a hereditary sensorimotor neuropathy or in postpolio syndrome. In addition, it may occur secondarily to trauma to the lateral capsular structures of the first MTPJ or to the attenuation of the joint capsule secondary to inflammatory joint diseases. However, the most common cause of hallux varus is iatrogenic, particularly after corrective surgery for hallux valgus, with a reported incidence varying from 2% to 13%.[1–3] There is a strong preponderance in women, with a mean age at presentation of 45 to 50 years.[4,5] Patients may complain of pain, difficulty with fitting footwear, unacceptable cosmesis, or functional impairment with associated instability and weak toe pushoff.[6–9] Some investigators have noted that the deformity can be well tolerated by patients over the longer term.[10]

Historically, the McBride procedure has been frequently implicated because of the destabilizing effects of releasing the insertion of the adductor hallucis, often in conjunction with excision of the lateral sesamoid.[6–8,11–14] This process causes the varus deformity as a consequence of the unopposed pull of abductor hallucis together

Sheffield Foot and Ankle Unit, Department of Trauma & Orthopaedic Surgery, Sheffield Teaching Hospitals NHS Foundation Trust, Herries Road, Sheffield S5 7AU, UK
* Corresponding author.
E-mail address: mark.davies@sth.nhs.uk

Foot Ankle Clin N Am 19 (2014) 275–284
http://dx.doi.org/10.1016/j.fcl.2014.02.010
1083-7515/14/$ – see front matter © 2014 Elsevier Inc. All rights reserved.

with the medial head of flexor hallucis brevis. Further imbalance of the toe extensors and the flexor hallucis longus can lead to a hyperextension deformity at the first MTPJ with a flexion deformity of the interphalangeal joint (IPJ). Other documented surgical procedures that have led to iatrogenic hallux varus as a complication include Keller-Brandes,[6,8,10,11] scarf,[3,14] Petersen,[8,13] distal,[6,15] and basal osteotomies,[10,16] and the Lapidus procedure.[17] Other than McBride procedures, essentially any excessive resection of the medial eminence, overcorrection of intermetatarsal angle with an osteotomy, release of the lateral soft tissues, or plication of the medial tissues in any combination risks the development of hallux varus.

CLASSIFICATION AND TREATMENT

An ideal classification system acts as a reliable and reproducible tool that can be used both practically, in terms of an accompanying treatment algorithm, and in terms of permitting comparable groups for research. However, for iatrogenic hallux varus no such classification exists, as each deformity is uniquely dependent on the degree and nature of the iatrogenic insult. Donley[18] attempted to classify acquired hallux varus in 2 ways: firstly by dividing hallux varus into static and dynamic deformities, and secondly by considering the axial and sagittal plane deformities at both the MTPJ and the IPJ. However, this article considered all causes of acquired hallux varus rather than focusing on iatrogenic causes. Similarly, classifying hallux varus according to whether the deformities are fixed or flexible may be oversimplistic, particularly when there is a wide variety of surgical treatment described within the literature.[9] Previously described surgical guidelines[9] and treatment algorithms[6] are not easy to follow, and may not include all treatment options for every individual scenario.

An attempt has been made to specifically classify the etiology of iatrogenic hallux varus into 4 distinct groups by the underlying dominant surgical insult responsible for the deformity.[8] This classification is possibly an oversimplification, especially in the presence of a combination of causes, and therefore a treatment algorithm may not be applicable.

CLINICAL EXAMINATION AND INVESTIGATION

Inspection of the patient's foot while standing and bearing weight reveals the severity of the varus deformity at the first MTPJ. In addition, deformity at the IPJ can be observed as well as any associated hyperextension or rotation at the first MTPJ. Other information such as previous surgical wounds and the health of the soft-tissue integumen can also be ascertained.

With the patient seated, the first MTPJ and IPJ can be assessed for fixity, flexibility, reducibility, discomfort, and crepitus. Flexible and reducible deformities may be considered for joint-preserving surgical treatments, whereas painful and stiff joints with crepitus may be best treated with arthrodeses.

Plain orthogonal standing radiographs demonstrate the health of the first MTPJ and IPJ including congruency. In addition, sequential plain films may reveal progressive joint destruction and osteomyelitis as the cause of iatrogenic hallux varus in cases of suspected deep sepsis. Magnetic resonance imaging may help determine the extent of infection in these latter cases, and can have a role in suspected avascular necrosis of the first metatarsal head.

NONOPERATIVE TREATMENT

It is accepted that early recognition of iatrogenic hallux varus allows the surgeon a window of opportunity to manage the deformity without the need for further surgery.[6,7]

Important factors determining a successful outcome from nonoperative treatment include the degree and flexibility of the deformity. Beverage and Leemrijse[9] state that at least 3 months of taping the hallux in a corrected position may lead to a successful outcome. Skalley and Myerson[6] observed that 22% of their series of 54 patients had moderately successful outcomes following taping, splintage, wide toe-box footwear, and nonsteroidal anti-inflammatory medication. Although the degree of varus deformity does not correlate with a poor outcome, Trnka and colleagues[10] noted that in the main, a deformity greater than 15° varus is associated with patient dissatisfaction.

OPERATIVE TREATMENTS
Soft-Tissue Rebalancing

For patients in whom the primary deformity is due to excessive plication of the medial capsule and ligamentous structures, and in the absence of any joint contracture, repair and plication of the lateral joint capsule is seldom effective. However, release of the medial capsule combined with abductor hallucis tenotomy and postoperative splintage may be effective if recognized early,[7] but is rarely effective in severe deformities.[6]

Tendon Transfer Procedures

The operative aim in correcting flexible and passively correctable hallux varus is to try to redress the tendon imbalance of the motors crossing the first MTPJ. Hawkins[19] presented the long-term outcome of surgical treatment of 3 cases of hallux varus following a McBride procedure. He described detaching the abductor hallucis tendon from the base of the proximal phalanx and transferring it plantar to the first metatarsal and deep to the intermetatarsal ligament, to insert it through a bone tunnel from the lateral aspect of the proximal phalanx and secure it with a suture. Although this technique has been attempted by many investigators, there are technical challenges of achieving sufficient tendon length to transfer, and residual supination of the toe may occur as a result of the plantar attachment of the transferred tendon.[14]

Johnson and Spiegl[11] were keen to devise a more dynamic tendon transfer procedure, and in 1984 described a new technique and the results in 15 feet. The whole of the extensor hallucis longus (EHL) tendon is detached from the insertion, then routed plantar to the intermetatarsal ligament and inserted into the lateral aspect of the base of the proximal phalanx. In addition, the IPJ is arthrodesed to prevent a flexion deformity of this joint. Johnson subsequently modified this procedure by performing a split EHL transfer (4 patients) to avoid IPJ arthrodesis in those individuals without IPJ contracture.[7] Goldman and colleagues[12] reviewed 9 patients with iatrogenic hallux varus treated either with a complete EHL transfer with IPJ arthrodesis (5 patients) or a split EHL transfer, with a mean follow-up of 20 months. Eight of the 9 patients were completely satisfied with the results of the surgery, including one individual who was corrected into valgus, one who had a resting plantarflexion deformity of the hallux, and one with neurogenic pain. The dissatisfied patient had recurrent hallux varus caused by a fracture through the osseous tunnel in the proximal phalanx where the EHL transfer was secured.

Dissatisfaction with the Hawkins tendon transfer (owing to the lack of sufficient tendon length to transfer) and the Johnson technique (with the desire to preserve IPJ motion and avoid passing EHL through scarred intermetatarsal tissues) led Leemrijse and colleagues[14] to devise a new tendon transfer technique termed the "reverse" Hawkins transfer. The aim of this transfer is to reconstruct the lateral collateral ligament. The medial capsule is released and the abductor hallucis tendon is detached proximally so as to maintain the attachment to the proximal phalanx. The tendon is then passed through a tunnel in the proximal phalangeal base into the first web space. Once there, it is then passed deep to the intermetatarsal ligament, then passed through a drill hole into the first metatarsal neck and secured there. In a 2-year follow-up of 7 cases of iatrogenic hallux varus following a mixture of McBride and scarf procedures, no complications were noted, and all patients had improved American Orthopaedic Foot and Ankle Society scores and were able to wear off-the-shelf footwear.[14]

In an attempt to improve the scientific level of evidence for the use of tendon transfer surgery for treating flexible iatrogenic hallux varus, Plovanich and colleagues[5] conducted a systematic review of the literature. Eight studies (7 level IV evidence and 1 level V evidence) were included, which identified 52 patients (68 feet). Forty-one feet were treated with the Johnson technique, 9 with Hawkins transfers, 7 with a modified reverse Hawkins technique, 7 with a first dorsal interosseous transfer,[20] and 4 with an extensor hallucis brevis (EHB) tenodesis.[21] With a mean follow-up of 30 months, this study concluded that tendon transfer surgery afforded an acceptable treatment option for flexible iatrogenic hallux varus in the short term, but noted a 16.2% complication rate. Complications consisted of first MTPJ degenerative change in 5.9%, recurrent hallux varus in 4.4% (only in cases treated with a Johnson transfer), hallux valgus in 2.9%, valgus and complex regional pain syndrome, and first intermetatarsal space neuritis.

Tenodeses

Skalley and Myerson[6] gained experience with the split EHL transfer technique, but noted that the technique was more difficult in patients with scarring around the EHL tendon. As a result, a static tenodesis procedure using EHB was devised as an alternative.[21] In this technique, the EHB is detached proximally and mobilized back to the insertion on the extensor hood. It is then routed deep to the intermetatarsal ligament and secured to the first metatarsal head under sufficient tension to correct the deformity and to maintain an acceptable range of first MTPJ motion (**Fig. 1**). In all 6 cases the outcomes were excellent. Furthermore, Lau and Myerson[22] noted that with split EHL transfer techniques, the transferred half of EHL is noted to bowstring during tensioning. Therefore, an alternative tenodesis was described whereby the lateral half of the EHL tendon is detached proximally and routed deep to the intermetatarsal ligament before being sutured back onto itself with appropriate tension to correct the deformity and preserve motion of the great toe joints. A further case series, using a minimally invasive technique of transferring either the EHB or the lateral half of the EHL tendon to act as tenodeses in the same fashion as the open techniques, has been described in 5 cases, with the only noted complication of paresthesia in the lateral border of the great toe.[23]

Synthetic Ligamentous Reconstructive Procedures

The lateral collateral ligament can be reconstructed using synthetic materials. Tourne and colleagues[8] assessed the surgical treatment of two groups of patients with iatrogenic hallux varus, one with degenerative change at the first MTPJ that were treated with arthrodesis and another group with mobile, pain-free first MTPJ that proceeded to lateral collateral ligament reconstruction using a synthetic ligament material. Although the groups were not comparable, the outcomes following surgery were encouraging when assessed with an unvalidated 100-point scoring system. In the group of 9 cases treated with first MTPJ arthrodesis, 5 had an "excellent" and 4 had

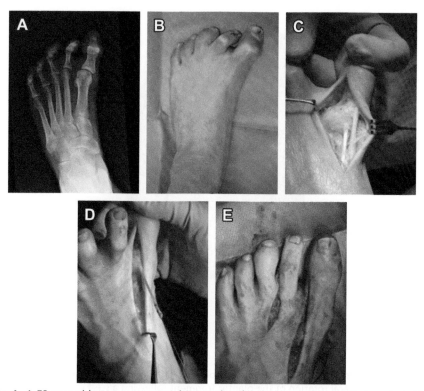

Fig. 1. A 52-year old woman presented 3 months after kicking a door while barefoot. She presented with a hallux varus deformity, a flexion deformity of the interphalangeal joint (IPJ), and a concurrent second hammertoe (*A, B*). All deformities were correctable. She underwent a medial capsular release and a tenodesis procedure using the extensor hallucis brevis (*C, D*) to correct the hallux varus deformity. The IPJ deformity was dynamic, and reduced with tensioning of the tenodesis. The second hammertoe was treated with a Weil osteotomy and plantar plate repair (*E*). (*Courtesy of* Mr H.G. Davies.)

a "good" outcome. Of the 5 cases treated with a lateral collateral ligament reconstruction, all achieved an "excellent" outcome.

More recently, 2 investigators independently advocated the use of mini suture–endobutton constructs for the surgical treatment of hallux varus wherein there is a primary soft-tissue imbalance that requires addressing.[24,25] In this technique, the Fibrewire suture is secured to the medial aspect of the metaphyseal-diaphyseal junction of the proximal phalanx with an endobutton and then passed through a drill hole in the first metatarsal neck, before the endobutton is snugged onto the medial cortex of the first metatarsal neck and the construct tensioned to correct the deformity. Given that these were isolated case reports with favorable outcomes using this reconstructive technique, there is insufficient evidence to recommend the use of such techniques.

Corrective Osteotomies

Excessive correction of the intermetatarsal angle has been defined as a resultant intermetatarsal angle of between less than 0°[9] and less than 2° (**Fig. 2**).[26] Following excessive reduction of the intermetatarsal angle, in conjunction with soft-tissue procedures, one approach to treat the hallux varus is to correct the deformity by performing

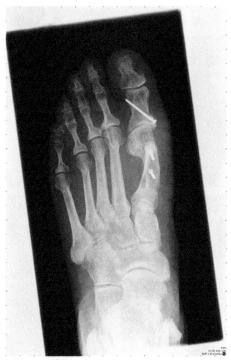

Fig. 2. Plain radiograph of a 70-year old woman with excessive resection of the medial eminence and lateral rotation of the plantar fragment following a scarf osteotomy, leaving a clinically tolerated mild hallux varus deformity.

corrective osteotomies. Until recently within the literature, experience of salvage osteotomies has been confined to either isolated case reports,[27] small case series,[6,28] or technical tips,[29] with no clear evidence of surgical outcomes. Correction of iatrogenic hallux varus following scarf osteotomy by reosteotomizing and reversing the correction, with or without an opening wedge proximal phalangeal osteotomy, has been described in 4 patients to good effect.[30]

In 2011, Choi and colleagues[4] published the largest experience of corrective distal metatarsal osteotomies for iatrogenic hallux varus. In this study, approximately two-thirds of the 19 patients reviewed had been treated for hallux valgus with scarf osteotomies and the remainder with a proximal chevron osteotomy. All had concurrent Akin osteotomies. The corrective osteotomy used in all cases was a 60° angled distal chevron osteotomy, creating a distal fragment that was medialized by 4 to 5 mm before an additional biplanar medial closing wedge osteotomy was performed to correct the distal metatarsal articular angle. Additional lateral capsular plication was required in some cases. In 90% of the patients, a significant improvement was achieved in the radiologic parameters, and even though 2 of the 19 patients had recurrence of their hallux varus deformities, only 1 patient remained dissatisfied with the outcome of the procedure.

Reconstruction of the Medial Eminence of First Metatarsal Head

In those cases where the hallux varus seems to be largely due to excessive resection of the medial eminence of the first metatarsal head, and in the absence of a painful, stiff, or arthritic first MTPJ, reconstruction of the medial eminence has been advocated. Rochwerger and colleagues[13] described the results of corrective surgery in 7 cases of symptomatic hallux varus secondary to aggressive resection of the medial eminence. The bone loss was replaced by exposing the medial aspect of the first metatarsal head, and lagging and sculpting a piece of autologous iliac crest to the metatarsal head. It is

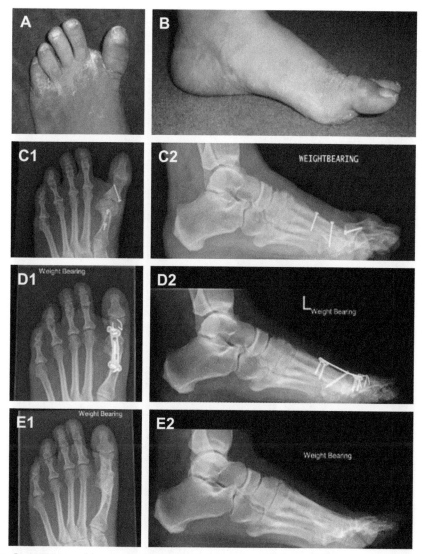

Fig. 3. A 50-year old woman presented to the authors with a painful, rigid hallux varus deformity and an inability to wear a shoe with an enclosed toe box (*A*). Fifteen years previously, she had undergone a Mitchell procedure to correct her hallux valgus deformity. Unfortunately, she was unhappy with the outcome of surgery as she had a persistent, painful hallux valgus deformity, so she underwent a revision procedure using scarf and Akin osteotomies that resulted in the hallux varus deformity (*B*). In addition, there was a fixed flexion deformity of the IPJ. The patient underwent a first metatarsophalangeal joint (MTPJ) arthrodesis using a dorsal locking plate and an additional dorsal closing wedge osteotomy to the distal phalanx secured with 2 staples (*C, D*). After subsequent metalwork removal, she was pleased with the result and was able to wear off-the-shelf enclosed footwear (*E*).

unclear from this study whether additional soft-tissue balancing, particularly of the adductor hallucis tendon, other than a medial soft-tissue release was required.

One of the 7 cases was dissatisfied with the results because of perceived overcorrection into valgus.

Arthrodesis

Hallux varus in the presence of articular destruction or an irreducible, stiff first MTPJ invariably necessitates arthrodesis of the first MTPJ, and remains the ultimate salvage

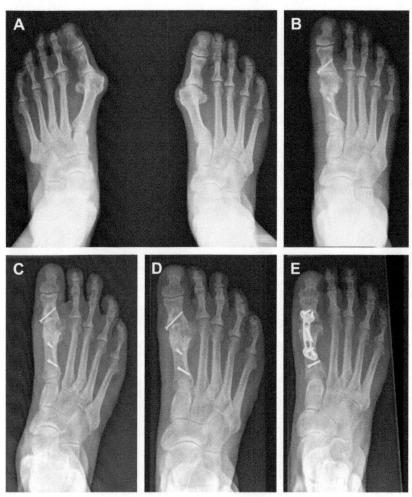

Fig. 4. A 73-year old woman presented with persistent pain around her first MTPJ a year after right-sided scarf and Akin osteotomies for a hallux valgus deformity (*A, B*). She had experienced a wound dehiscence and received multiple oral antibiotic courses in that year. Serial plain radiographs showed the progressive destruction of the first MTPJ and a worsening hallux varus deformity (*C, D*). The IPJ exhibited a full range of motion. As a primary investigation, the screw was removed from the proximal phalanx, and bone biopsies were taken from the proximal phalanx and the metatarsal head. This screw grew a coagulase-negative *Staphylococcus aureus* sensitive to flucloxacillin. Subsequently a first metatarsophalangeal arthrodesis was performed with flucloxacillin treatment perioperatively (*E*).

procedure.[6–8] The only difficult caveat to this is the concurrent degeneration, contracture, or stiffness of the IPJ (**Fig. 3**). Arthrodesis of both the first MTPJ and the IPJ can be performed provided that there is a degree of shortening of the first ray so as to reduce the lever arm on the toe.[7] Intuitively it is preferable to preserve the IPJ so that arthrodesis of the first MTPJ may be combined with arthrolysis of the IPJ[9] or a phalangeal osteotomy to reorientate the arc of motion within the IPJ (see **Fig. 3**).

It is also prudent to consider that rapid degeneration of the first MTPJ in the presence of hallux varus may be secondary to overzealous surgical techniques and also to deep joint infection. Any history of delayed wound healing and repeated use of postoperative antibiotics should be considered when assessing the patient. Before planning corrective surgery, deep tissue biopsies should be taken after a suitable period of abstinence from antibiotic therapy. Any organisms grown can then be targeted with perioperative antibiotic therapy, and it may be necessary for staged arthrodesis in certain circumstances (**Fig. 4**).

SUMMARY

The most common cause of hallux varus, an uncommon outcome of hallux surgery that may be well tolerated, is iatrogenic. There are no good classifications because the condition has such varied surgical etiology. In terms of treatment, management may be nonoperative, although expert opinion suggests that the role of this is limited. Surgical management by way of simple soft-tissue releases is unlikely to be effective if undertaken as isolated procedures, with the possible exception of mild deformities that have been detected early. A large range of complex soft-tissue transfers have been described, with small series reporting fair results. Bony corrections have also been described, mostly as small case series. In the presence of joint degeneration or a history of infection, the authors would advocate that the presence of deep infection is excluded. Arthrodesis remains the most predictable salvage procedure for the treatment of iatrogenic hallux varus.

REFERENCES

1. Peterson DA, Zilberfarb JL, Greene MA, et al. Avascular necrosis of the first metatarsal head: incidence in distal osteotomy combined with lateral soft tissue release. Foot Ankle Int 1994;15:59–63.
2. Hansen CE. Hallux valgus treated by the McBride operation. Acta Orthop Scand 1974;45:778–92.
3. Kilmartin TE, O'Kane C. Combined rotation scarf and Akin osteotomies for hallux valgus: a patient focussed 9 year follow up of 50 patients. J Foot Ankle Res 2010; 3:2.
4. Choi KJ, Lee HS, Yoon YS, et al. Distal metatarsal osteotomy for hallux varus following surgery for hallux valgus. J Bone Joint Surg Br 2011;93:1079–83.
5. Plovanich EJ, Donnenwerth MP, Abicht BP, et al. Failure after soft-tissue release with tendon transfer for flexible iatrogenic hallux varus: a systematic review. J Foot Ankle Surg 2012;51:195–7.
6. Skalley TC, Myerson MS. The operative treatment of acquired hallux varus. Clin Orthop Relat Res 1994;306:183–91.
7. Coughlin MJ, Mann RA. Surgery of the foot and ankle. 7th edition. St Louis (MO): Mosby; 1999. p. 258–66.
8. Tourne Y, Saragaglia D, Picard F, et al. Iatrogenic hallux varus surgical procedure: a study of 14 cases. Foot Ankle Int 1995;16:457–63.

9. Bevernage BD, Leemrijse T. Hallux varus: classification and treatment. Foot Ankle Clin 2009;14:51–65.

10. Trnka HJ, Zettl R, Hungerford M, et al. Acquired hallux varus and clinical tolerability. Foot Ankle Int 1997;18:593–7.

11. Johnson KA, Spiegl PV. Extensor hallucis longus transfer for hallux varus deformity. J Bone Joint Surg Am 1984;66:681–6.

12. Goldman FD, Siegel J, Barton E. Extensor hallucis longus tendon transfer for correction of hallux varus. J Foot Ankle Surg 1993;32:126–31.

13. Rochwerger A, Curvale G, Groulier P. Application of bone graft to the medial side of the first metatarsal head in the treatment of hallux varus. J Bone Joint Surg Am 1999;81:1730–5.

14. Leemrijse T, Hoang B, Maldague P, et al. A new surgical procedure for iatrogenic hallux varus: reverse transfer of the abductor hallucis tendon. A report of 7 cases. Acta Orthop Belg 2008;74:227–34.

15. Pochatko DJ, Schlehr FJ, Murphey MD, et al. Distal chevron osteotomy with lateral release for treatment of hallux valgus deformity. Foot Ankle Int 1994;15:457–61.

16. Mann RA, Rudicel S, Graves SC. Repair of hallux valgus with a distal soft tissue procedure and proximal metatarsal osteotomy. J Bone Joint Surg Am 1992;74:124–9.

17. Mauldin DM, Sanders M, Whitmer WW. Correction of hallux valgus with metatarsocuneiform stabilization. Foot Ankle Int 1990;11:59–66.

18. Donley BG. Acquired hallux varus. Foot Ankle Int 1997;18:586–92.

19. Hawkins FB. Acquired hallux varus: cause, prevention and correction. Clin Orthop Relat Res 1971;76:169–76.

20. Valtin B. First dorsal interosseous muscle transfer in iatrogenic hallux varus. Med Chir Pied 1991;7:9–16 [in French].

21. Myerson MS, Komenda GA. Results of hallux varus correction using an extensor hallucis brevis tenodesis. Foot Ankle Int 1996;17:21–7.

22. Lau JTC, Myerson MS. Modified split extensor hallucis longus tendon transfer for correction of hallux varus. Foot Ankle Int 2002;32:1138–40.

23. Lui TH. Technique tip: minimally invasive approach of tendon transfer for correction of hallux varus. Foot Ankle Int 2009;30:1018–21.

24. Gerbert J, Traynor C, Blue K, et al. Use of Mini Tightrope for correction of hallux varus deformity. J Foot Ankle Surg 2011;50:245–51.

25. Hsu AR, Gross CE, Lin JL. Bilateral hallux varus deformity correction with a suture button construct. Am J Orthop 2013;42:121–4.

26. Belczyk R, Stapleton JJ, Grossman JP, et al. Complications and revisional hallux valgus surgery. Clin Podiatr Med Surg 2009;26:475–84.

27. Bilotti MA, Caprioli R, Testa J, et al. Reverse Austin osteotomy for correction of hallux varus. J Foot Surg 1987;26:51–6.

28. Zahari DT, Girolamo M. Hallux varus: a step wise approach for correction. J Foot Surg 1991;30:264–6.

29. Lee KT, Park YU, Young KW, et al. Reverse distal chevron osteotomy to treat iatrogenic hallux varus after overcorrection of the intermetatarsal 1-2 angle: technical tip. Foot Ankle Int 2011;32:89–91.

30. Kannegieter E, Kilmartin TE. The combined reverse scarf and opening wedge osteotomy of the proximal phalanx for the treatment of iatrogenic hallux varus. Foot 2011;21:88–91.

Transfer Metatarsalgia Post Hallux Valgus Surgery

Ernesto Maceira, MD[a,b], Manuel Monteagudo, MD[a,b],*

KEYWORDS

- Metatarsalgia • Hallux valgus • Metatarsal osteotomy • Weil osteotomy • Forefoot

KEY POINTS

- No surgical procedure in hallux valgus surgery is free of complications. Metatarsalgia may arise because of iatrogenic mechanical impairments.
- Identification and hierarchization of the mechanical impairments involved in a particular case is critical to eliminate pain and restore foot function as much as possible.
- Surgical management of metatarsalgia may require surgical procedures in different anatomic regions other than the forefoot.
- Functional or anatomic equinus is important during the second and the early third rocker but not at the late propulsive phase.
- Metatarsal length is important in the third rocker pathologic abnormality but not in the second rocker overload.
- Patients may present with combined second and third rocker pathologic abnormality at a given ray or at different rays.
- There are several "what should not be done" items that may be useful in the surgical planning of mechanical metatarsalgia, as follows:
  - Do not shorten a metatarsal with evidence of second rocker overload (second rocker keratosis, extensor over recruitment). Otherwise, overloading will persist and the toe will develop additional dorsiflexion contracture.
  - Do not elevate a metatarsal with evidence of third rocker overload (third rocker keratosis, MP joint instability). Otherwise, a central ray insufficiency syndrome may develop with second rocker overload at the neighbor rays.
  - Do not lengthen the gastrocnemius in the absence of gastrocnemius-dependent equinus, as is the case in pure third rocker pathologic abnormality.
- The order of priorities in foot surgery is to achieve a pain-free, plantigrade, and flexible foot.

---

[a] Faculty of Medicine, Universidad Europea Madrid, Calle Diego De Velazquez, 28223 Pozuelo De Alarcon, Madrid, Spain; [b] Orthopaedic Foot and Ankle Unit, Orthopaedic and Trauma Department, Hospital Universitario Quirón Madrid, Madrid, Spain
* Corresponding author.
E-mail address: mmontyr@yahoo.com

Foot Ankle Clin N Am 19 (2014) 285–307
http://dx.doi.org/10.1016/j.fcl.2014.03.001
1083-7515/14/$ – see front matter © 2014 Elsevier Inc. All rights reserved.

INTRODUCTION

Reconstructive hallux valgus surgery is one of the most common procedures in foot and ankle practice. Some cases develop a painful hallux with malposition postoperatively. When there is no metatarsalgia (or even in moderately painful metatarsalgia with an adequate metatarsal parabola), repositioning of the first ray may be enough to achieve a pain-free forefoot. Unfortunately, other complications of hallux valgus surgery may develop. Common complications include undercorrection or recurrence, overcorrection or hallux varus, shortening, nonunion, and malunion with elevation (dorsiflexion) or with plantarflexion of the first metatarsal. Sometimes these complications may be asymptomatic but frequently render a first metatarsal that is unable to function properly. If the first ray cannot bear much of the body weight during the second and third rockers of gait (forefoot contact to toe off), a shift of plantar pressures to the lesser metatarsals may occur. Iatrogenic transfer metatarsalgia is more prevalent than previously thought and incidence is possibly increasing.[1,2] In most cases dysfunction after a failed hallux valgus surgery is the cause of lesser metatarsals overload, but failure to achieve the right metatarsal parabola or malalignment of a lesser metatarsal osteotomy can also cause transfer metatarsalgia of the adjacent metatarsals.

Between 11% and 20% of patients develop transfer metatarsalgia following Mitchell osteotomy. Recurrence of the deformity and shortening of the first metatarsal are the most common causes of transfer metatarsalgia.[3–5]

Management of transfer metatarsalgia after hallux valgus surgery is challenging to the experienced foot and ankle surgeon. A thorough understanding of the pathomechanics underlying the failed hallux is fundamental to plan the proper treatment. A detailed history and clinical examination together with image studies will allow the determination of what went wrong and why. If conservative measures fail to relieve pain, revision surgery may be indicated. In some cases, a successful outcome may be expected from revision of the first ray, but in other cases, surgery on the lesser rays or both combined may be necessary to achieve a mechanically sound forefoot.

Excluded in this work is discussion of other complications of hallux valgus surgery that may cause transfer metatarsalgia: hematoma, nerve injury, complex regional pain syndrome, trauma, skin problems surrounding the first ray, infection, and thrombophlebitis. Discussion is concentrated on addressing pathomechanics, clinical examination, image studies, and conservative surgical management of first ray and the lesser rays for the treatment of transfer metatarsalgia.

PATHOMECHANICS

The term transfer metatarsalgia refers to the onset of pain at a different ray than that which is mechanically impaired. Malfunction of a given metatarsophalangeal (MP) joint may produce pain at another MP joint. Hallux valgus surgery may impair first ray function and produce signs and symptoms at any other region around the lesser MP joints.[6,7]

Continuous mechanical overload leading to tissue stress may turn biologic damage symptomatic. Any tissue can suffer the consequences of compressive, tensile, or shearing stress.[8] Metatarsal stress fractures are well-known examples of injuries produced by cyclic loading. Osteoarthritis (of biomechanical origin) of the first MP joint is the end result of abnormal loading of the articular surfaces due to rolling contact instead of the physiologic gliding contact pattern that should take place at that joint. Iatrogenic stiffness of the first MP joint can precipitate arthritis. Plantar plate rupture (of biomechanical origin) is the end result of abnormal cyclic loading on the plantar-distal region of a lesser MP joint. The plantar fat pad undergoes atrophic changes because of cyclic loading, but the skin hypertrophies, generating keratoses that show different patterns depending on the location and kind of stress, either compressive or shearing (**Fig. 1**).

By studying the consequences of tissue stress, the surgeon must try to identify as accurately as possible which of the main causative factors are producing transfer metatarsalgia, as well as their hierarchical importance.[9]

FOREFOOT, METATARSALGIA, AND GAIT

In this article, the "rockers" from gait analysis are referred to so as to understand the pathomechanics of transfer metatarsalgia.[10] The contact pattern between the foot and the ground varies during the stance phase. The tibia keeps on rotating forward throughout the stance. A rocking point for the tibia to rotate is needed along the stance phase to achieve simultaneous continuous progression and stability.[11]

During the *first rocker*, the tibia rotates on the heel, which is the only part of the sole of the foot contacting the ground. Obviously, there is no compressive stress on the plantar structures of the forefoot during this rocker. However, abnormal forces, such as the action of extensor tendons' over-recruitment, can take place during the heel rocker and swing phase if the tibialis anterior and peroneus tertius are unable to cope with plantar flexing moments at the ankle around initial contact. The toes may claw because of these compensatory mechanisms to oppose equinus.

As soon as the forefoot contacts the ground, the tibia can no longer rotate on the heel and starts rotating onto the talus. The foot-ground contact pattern during the *second (ankle) rocker* is plantigrade. Although the weight-bearing (WB) limb is the only one supporting the body, its contact pattern with the ground is the most stable. Any mechanical overload at a given metatarsal head during the second rocker will stress the soft tissues located strictly plantar to the metatarsal head due to the vertical, compressive stress during the second rocker. The metatarsal bones must support dorsiflexing moments during this rocker and this can finally result in stress fracture at the neck of the metatarsal. There is no foot rotation on the ground during this rocker: the foot is plantigrade and the external rotation of the leg is entirely performed on the foot skeleton. Second rocker keratoses tend to be discrete, making it quite easy to determine which keratosis

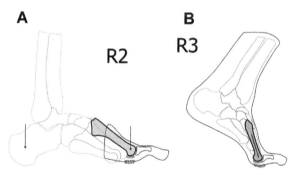

Fig. 1. Pathomechanics of metatarsalgia. (*A*) During the second rocker (R2), the contact pattern is plantrigrade. Ground reaction forces are vertically applied strictly beneath the metatarsal head. The heel supports weight as well and the plantar plate is quite safe. (*B*) During the third rocker (R3), the foot is vertically oriented on the ground. The forefoot represents only the contact area of the supporting limb. Load is transmitted axially through the metatarsal long axis. Soft tissue stress will be suffered by the plantar plate at its distal end and by the skin located in a planto-distal position relative to the metatarsal head.

is produced by which metatarsal. The plantar plate is usually not injured during this rocker, because part of the body weight is supported by the hindfoot.

Metatarsal length is not relevant during static stance or mid stance, while the foot is plantigrade on the ground. Mechanical impairments that may overload the forefoot during plantigrade support are anatomic plantarflexion of one or more metatarsals (ie, pes cavus, plantarflexed metatarsal), elevation of an adjacent metatarsal (such as iatrogenic metatarsal elevation), and increased plantarflexor moment at the ankle joint (equinus deformity). Because gastrocnemius tension is dependent on the position of the knee (tight with extended knee, relaxed with knee flexion), contracture of the elastic component of the gastrocnemius can overload the forefoot during the second rocker and the transition from second to third rocker, when the knee should be in extension. Gastrocnemius cannot be responsible for forefoot overloading at the late third rocker, because both the knee and the ankle are flexed by that time.

Transition from the second to the *third rocker* starts at heel lift, because, at that point, the body weight is supported just at the forefoot. Because of the triceps surae, the third rocker or propulsive phase allows for the body center of mass to elevate, increasing potential energy. The ankle undergoes progressive plantarflexion and the longitudinal axis of the foot is placed vertically on the ground. Dorsiflexion at the MP break line, together with appropriate relative metatarsal length and plantarflexion of the first metatarsal, provides for balanced distribution of compressive axial forces throughout the metatarsal heads, from lateral to medial. Extrinsic muscles of the foot and the plantar aponeurosis play an important role in keeping adequate alignment between the leg, ankle, heel, and forefoot during this phase. Iatrogenic lack of first MP dorsiflexion may block progression on the sagittal plane, thus requiring compensatory mechanisms that may eventually result in first and/or lesser ray overloading. One of the compensatory mechanisms for an iatrogenic hallux limitus can be foot supination during the third rocker, which would stress the lateral rays.[1]

Metatarsal bones also suffer stress during the third rocker. Axial loading while the metatarsal is vertically aligned on the ground compresses equally both compact and cancellous bone. Because most of the metatarsal head is made out of cancellous bone and its elastic modulus is lower than that of compact bone, a transverse fracture may occur at the head itself, impairing blood flow at the tip of the metatarsal and producing secondary osteonecrosis (Freiberg disease). The authors think that collapse of the metatarsal head shortens the bone, up to the point needed to achieve an ideal metatarsal parabola.

Metatarsal length is important during the third rocker. It is the most significant cause of propulsive metatarsalgia. The ideal metatarsal parabola is that which allows for an even distribution of axial loading on all of the metatarsal heads during propulsion, without the need for participation of active elements. All of the metatarsal radiographic variants are normal as long as the foot is painless and functional. They should be considered pathologic when symptoms develop. For example, an iatrogenic index minus foot (first metatarsal shorter than the second one) will be functional as long as some forces pull the first metatarsal downwards enough to let it purchase the ground. The active element responsible for generating a plantarflexor moment at the first tarsometatarsal joint is the peroneus longus. Despite the strength of the muscle, an effective moment arm is required for the tendon to depress the first metatarsal head effectively by pulling the first metatarsal base laterally and downwards. Hindfoot pronation, a deformity favored by gravity and aging, will decrease the plantarflexor component and increase the abduction component of the tendon function; if the first ray is unable to cope with medial support of the foot in the propulsive phase, force will be transferred to the central rays with potential pathologic consequences.[12,13]

CLINICAL EXAMINATION

Examining (or "reading") the sole of the foot provides valuable information regarding transfer metatarsalgia pathomechanics. Plantar skin is the best baropodometric record. Increased pressure and shear stress are responsible for the development of plantar callosities. The morphology of plantar keratoses reflects the contact pattern between the foot and the ground. Keratoses located strictly plantar to the metatarsal head(s) must be produced while the foot is plantigrade (during the second rocker or during static standing) and can be due to a true or relatively increased metatarsal pitch angle, a block to ankle dorsiflexion, or a gastrocnemius contracture.

Soft tissues that suffer stress during the third rocker are those located planto-distal to the metatarsal head(s), because the foot is not flat on the ground, but the heel is lifted during the propulsive phase (**Fig. 2**). Metatarsal length is obviously a significant factor in these callosities.

The presence of a second rocker keratosis under a metatarsal head can be due to functional or anatomic descent of the corresponding metatarsal, or to functional or anatomic elevation of an adjacent metatarsal. The presence of a third rocker keratosis under a metatarsal can be due to the excessive length of the corresponding metatarsal or to shortening of an adjacent metatarsal. Mixed second-third rocker callosities are especially common in the presence of transfer metatarsalgia after hallux valgus surgery.

It is therefore paramount that a thorough examination of plantar callosities is undertaken to determine the biomechanical cause of transfer metatarsalgia.

RADIOLOGICAL EVALUATION

Radiographic evaluation of the patient with transfer metatarsalgia after hallux valgus surgery should include WB dorsoplantar and lateral and oblique non-WB views. To estimate deformities and malunions of the first ray and its relationship with the lesser metatarsals, WB radiographs should be technically accurate so that accurate measurements can be made. A true WB radiograph of both feet will show the second metatarsocuneiform joint in orthogonal projection (**Fig. 3**). A true WB dorsoplantar view will allow one to draw a metatarsal parabola as reference for measurements and preoperative planning. The authors use a sheet of tracing paper to address the forefoot and determine their surgical strategy. There should be a geometric regression from the first to the fifth metatarsal. Ideally, the length of the first metatarsal should be equal or slightly shorter than the second metatarsal (index plus minus).[14] The Pedowitz classification allows the evaluation of the coverage of the sesamoids by the first metatarsal head.[15] Failure to reduce the first metatarsal over the sesamoids in hallux valgus surgery can produce first-ray mechanical failure and cause transfer metatarsalgia.[16] The amount of shortening for the lesser rays and hallux correction should be calculated over the WB radiographs (**Fig. 4**). Linear measurements, such as the relative lengths of the metatarsals, are reproducible and therefore useful for the preoperative planning of propulsive (third rocker) metatarsalgia, in the absence of tarsometatarsal deformities or dysfunction. Failure to restore proximal articular set angle (PASA) or distal metatarsal articular angle (DMAA) may also determine transfer metatarsalgia after surgical reconstruction of the hallux.

On the lateral view, the alignment of the first and second metatarsals can be addressed. In the nonoperated foot, the dorsal cortex of the diaphysis of both metatarsals should be parallel. A dorsiflexed or plantarflexed metatarsal can be identified. The amount of angular correction can be planned with this reference. Axial sesamoid

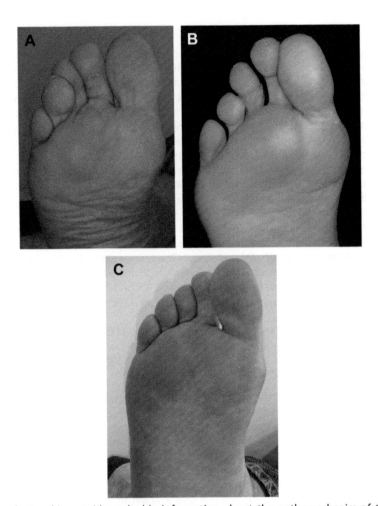

Fig. 2. Plantar skin provides valuable information about the pathomechanics of transfer metatarsalgia. (*A*) Second metatarsal elevation generating a second rocker keratosis underneath the third metatarsal. (*B*) Hallux valgus recurrence generating a third rocker keratosis. (*C*) Iatrogenic unloading of the first metatarsal. Notice the second rocker keratosis beneath the interphalangeal joint of the first toe and third rocker keratosis under the lesser metatarsals.

projection may be of help to estimate the position of the metatarsal head after surgery. Arthritic changes can also be evaluated.

Magnetic resonance imaging (MRI) may assist in determining the presence and extent of soft tissue, cartilage, and bone damage after hallux valgus surgery. MRI is also helpful to diagnose Freiberg disease, or a metatarsal stress fracture secondary to transfer metatarsalgia of the lesser rays. Computed tomography (CT) is of use for the evaluation of nonunions or malunions, loss of bone stock, subchondral cysts, osteophytes, sclerosis, and alteration in the normal contour of the metatarsal heads. In the future, the development of WB CT will be of great help in precisely calculating metatarsal lengths and angles for the evaluation and preoperative planning of transfer metatarsalgia.

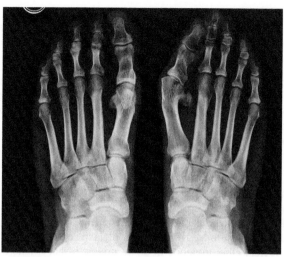

Fig. 3. A true dorsoplantar WB radiograph view shows the second metatarsocuneiform joint in orthogonal projection.

TREATMENT OF TRANSFER METATARSALGIA AFTER HALLUX VALGUS SURGERY
Conservative

Nonsurgical treatments should always be attempted for transfer metatarsalgia after hallux valgus surgery because they do not compromise future surgical revision. Treatment can include analgesics, offloading the painful joint or metatarsal head, padding, orthoses, adapted shoe modification, stretching exercises, and rocker-bottom shoes. There is no evidence to confirm the effectiveness of conservative measures for the

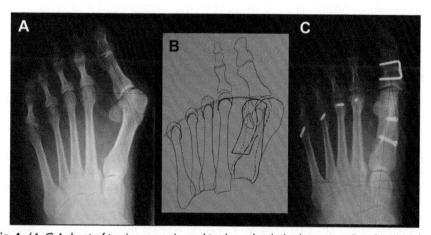

Fig. 4. (*A–C*) A sheet of tracing paper is used to draw the desired preoperative planning that includes reconstruction of the first ray and lesser metatarsals to restore a harmonic metatarsal parabola. The MSP (Barouk) was set 3 mm proximal to the previous level of the first metatarsal head to provide for adequate, tension-free reduction and realignment of the first MP joint. This means operating on all of the MP joints, an issue with which many authors disagree.

treatment of transfer metatarsalgia. However, some patients benefit from some of these therapies, especially those treatments with a mechanical basis (ie, orthoses, shoe modification).

Orthoses
Functional orthoses may be helpful to control abnormal hindfoot pronation or supination that might have an influence on transfer metatarsalgia. Accommodative insoles redistribute pressure under the forefoot. A metatarsal raise just proximal to lesser metatarsal heads on the insole or orthoses may distribute force away from the head of an excessively long metatarsal.[17]

Shoes
A wider toe box may relieve pain in patients with lesser toes deformities. Stretching the toe box overlying the first metatarsal head can also reduce pain in patients with hallux valgus recurrence. Lower heel height can help in some women suffering from transfer metatarsalgia. Rocker-bottom shoes seem to improve transition from the first to the third rocker and may alleviate transfer metatarsalgia in some patients.[18] Rocker soles are particularly useful in the presence of an iatrogenic hallux limitus or rigidus.

In some difficult cases, symptoms persist despite all efforts at nonoperative intervention; thus, revision surgery may be indicated.

Surgical
Surgical planning of transfer metatarsalgia after hallux valgus surgery starts by addressing the state of the first metatarsal. In many cases, revision surgery of the first ray will restore function and resolve lesser metatarsals overload.[19] If there is only shortening of the first metatarsal without elevation, shortening metatarsal osteotomies of the lesser rays will be used to achieve the right metatarsal parabola and reharmonize the metatarsal relative lengths.[20]

Gastrocnemius proximal release may be needed when a second rocker metatarsalgia is combined with a positive Silfverskiöld test.[21] Combined first and lesser rays procedures may be needed in some cases of transfer metatarsalgia after hallux valgus surgery.

First metatarsal
Of the possible surgical procedures for the first metatarsal, different scenarios can be considered.

First metatarsal nonunion Nonunion is a rare complication of first metatarsal osteotomies to correct hallux valgus. Most procedures are performed through metaphyseal bone, and fixation is used so healing is the expected result.[22] Nonunion after hallux valgus surgery may be due to biologic and biomechanical factors.

Biologic causes of nonunion usually result from an iatrogenic altered blood supply to the osteotomy site. No callus is observed and an atrophic nonunion develops. Diabetes, hypothyroidism, steroid intake, and hypoxia from anemia or cigarette smoking can lead to altered bone healing at an osteotomy site. During surgery, special care should be taken to respect blood supply to the first metatarsal, mainly at the plantar attachment of the MP joint capsule. Failure to respect these arteries may help to develop nonunion of the osteotomy and/or avascular necrosis of the first metatarsal head after hallux valgus surgery.[23]

Mechanical causes of nonunion are usually related to the osteotomy surgical technique. Proximal first metatarsal osteotomies are more unstable and more prone to nonunion, because there is an increased dorsiflexing moment arm through which loads are applied. Osteotomies with a single plane directed from dorsal proximal to plantar distal (ie, Ludloff) and those made perpendicular to the shaft of the first metatarsal (ie, closing abductory base wedge) are intrinsically unstable. Scarf osteotomy is intrinsically stable as long as the horizontal arm of the osteotomy is directed from dorsal distal to proximal plantar (ie, a long modified chevron). If the horizontal arm of a scarf osteotomy is made parallel to the longitudinal axis of the first metatarsal, troughing with elevation will possibly occur, and transfer metatarsalgia will be expected to develop.[24] Stable screw fixation is used for most first metatarsal osteotomies. The more inherently unstable the osteotomy, the more important the stability of fixation is. Most mechanical nonunions are hypertrophic with poor stability at the osteotomy site that allows for some motion. An incorrect placement of screws or an intraoperative fracture compromising the stability of the osteotomy may contribute to the development of a nonunion (**Fig. 5**).

Metatarsal nonunions after hallux valgus surgery are usually symptomatic and can result in a painful insufficient first ray that leads to transfer metatarsalgia. Management of nonunion can restore a mechanically sound first ray. In most cases, metalwork removal, debridement of the nonunion, bone grafting, realignment, and stable fixation will help to promote union.[25,26] The need for metatarsal surgery will depend on the preoperative planning once the ideal position of the first metatarsal over the sesamoids is determined. An altered metatarsal parabola may be an indication for a combined first and lesser metatarsal reconstruction procedure.

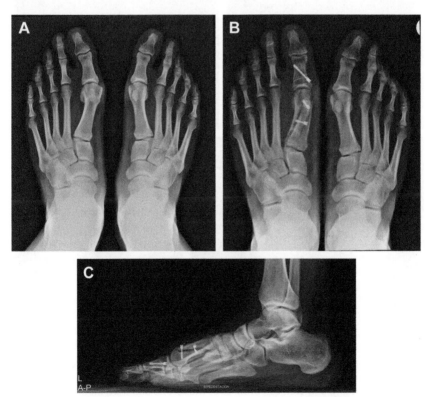

Fig. 5. Patient with painful hallux valgus. (*A*) Preoperative dorsoplantar view. (*B*) Postoperative dorsoplantar view. (*C*) Postoperative lateral view with broken screw, metatarsal elevation with fracture, and nonunion.

First metatarsal malunion

Undercorrection/Recurrence Undercorrection and recurrence of hallux valgus deformity after surgery has been reported as high as 16%.[7] An incomplete initial correction is possibly the most common explanation for recurrence. However, other factors may have an influence: ligamentous laxity, PASA, length of the first metatarsal, metatarsus adductus, medial column adductus, excessive hindfoot pronation, and ankle equinus contracture (that lead to hyperpronation) **(Fig. 6)**. Undercorrection and recurrence may be well tolerated with dissatisfaction arising from malalignment but is rarely true with metatarsalgia. Provided there is no first ray insufficiency from shortening nor elevation and metatarsal parabola is not seriously altered, undercorrection or recurrence may not produce transfer metatarsalgia. Commonly, however, deformity leads to mechanical overload of the lesser metatarsals and transfer metatarsalgia will have to be addressed.

Transfer metatarsalgia after undercorrection and recurrence should be treated by correcting the cause or causes of failure. Procedures will vary according to the

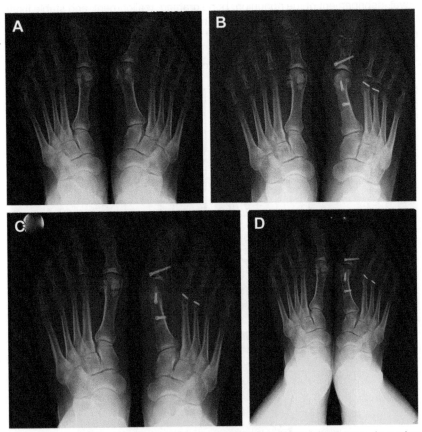

Fig. 6. Patient with painful hallux valgus and metatarsalgia. (*A*) Preoperative dorsoplantar WB view. (*B*) Four-week postoperative control after diaphyseal osteotomy of the first metatarsal, Akin osteotomy, and Weil osteotomies of the second and third metatarsals. An index plus has been iatrogenically generated. (*C*) Mild hallux valgus recurrence 1 year after surgery. (*D*) Two years after surgery, recurrence has been favored by an excessively long first metatarsal.

main problem observed and may include proximal medial gastrocnemius recession (gastrocnemius contracture), medial sliding calcaneal osteotomy (flexible flat foot deformity), cuneometatarsal arthrodesis (arthritis, ligamentous laxity, pronated foot), or a combination of several techniques.[27,28] In most cases, reconstruction of the first metatarsal is indicated. If cartilage in the first MP joint is severely damaged, fusion of the joint will be the option of choice; in these patients, there is no motion, or motion is painful during non-WB conditions. If not, an osteotomy should be performed to obtain adequate correction. Reduction of the first metatarsal head over the sesamoids, and restoration of PASA/DMAA balance, should be planned using preoperative WB radiographs. The metatarsal parabola should then be drawn and the need for shortening osteotomies of the lesser rays addressed. In the presence of transfer metatarsalgia and a correct metatarsal parabola after the projected first ray reconstruction on the preoperative planning, first metatarsal correction may be sufficient. If the metatarsal parabola reveals an excessive ideal length in one or more of the lesser metatarsals, shortening osteotomies should be included as part of the forefoot revision surgery planning. The article by Raikin and colleagues elsewhere in this issue deals with recurrent hallux valgus in depth.

Overcorrection/Hallux varus The incidence of hallux varus following hallux valgus surgery is reported to be as high as 12%.[7] Many patients with hallux varus are asymptomatic and do not need treatment, particularly in the absence of arthritis of the first MP joint and a mild deformity (<10°).[29] However, some patients present with metatarsalgia following an iatrogenic hallux varus deformity. An insufficient varus first ray in combination with a short first metatarsal leads to adduction of the lesser toes and the development of transfer metatarsalgia. Again, as in hallux valgus recurrence, special attention should be paid to the revision preoperative planning to address the need of lesser metatarsal osteotomies to restore the correct metatarsal parabola (**Fig. 7**). The article by Davies and Blundell elsewhere in this issue deals with iatrogenic hallux varus in depth.

Shortening Shortening of the first metatarsal has been well documented for various osteotomies.[3,30] The development of transfer metatarsalgia is a common finding in these patients. First ray insufficiency may cause overload of the central rays during the third rocker. Depending on how the lesser metatarsals cope with this overload, several scenarios may develop. A second metatarsal stress fracture will be the result of shortening and elevation of the first metatarsal head (ie, troughing in scarf osteotomy). Second space syndrome, with divergent second and third toes due to adduction at the second MP joint, can be due to an excessively long second metatarsal with respect to an iatrogenically shortened first metatarsal (**Fig. 8**). Frieberg disease is the result of abnormal axial metatarsal loading during the third rocker. A transverse cephalic stress fracture is followed by remodeling and dysplasia of the second metatarsal head. A long second metatarsal with respect to the shortened first metatarsal will impair the distal blood supply at the metatarsal head and facilitate collapse. In the presence of dysplasia, combined procedures over the second metatarsal head (ie, tilt-up osteotomy and triple Weil osteotomy) should be considered. Restoration of a harmonic metatarsal parabola should be the goal for surgical planning. Continuous repetitive stresses over the central metatarsals may cause injury to the plantar plate and, finally, an MP joint dislocation.[31] The article by Goldberg and Singh elsewhere in this issue deals with iatrogenic shortening of the first ray after hallux valgus surgery.

Elevation Elevation of the first metatarsal head can occur following a proximal, diaphyseal, or distal osteotomy.[32] Second and third metatarsals may develop a

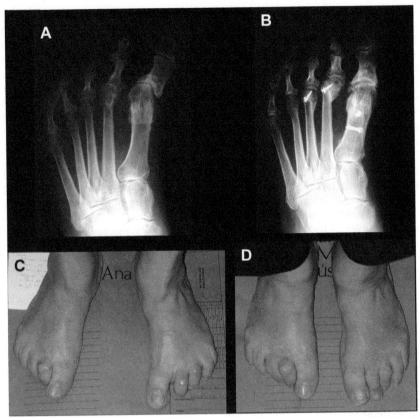

Fig. 7. Patient with hallux varus and transfer metatarsalgia after hallux valgus surgery. (*A*) Preoperative dorsoplantar radiograph for revision surgery planning. (*B*) Five-years postoperatively after reversed scarf and triple Weil osteotomies with medial cephalic gliding of the second and third metatarsals. (*C*) Preoperative clinical photo. (*D*) Five years postoperatively, the patient is asymptomatic and clinical correction is satisfactory.

second rocker overload and eventually a stress fracture of the second metatarsal. Midfoot pronation together with an iatrogenic hallux limitus may cause a third rocker overload at the fourth and fifth metatarsals. Elevation will cause the first MP joint to plantarflex to compensate for metatarsal elevation and the hallucal interphalangeal joint will dorsiflex to help with push-off at the third rocker. Traction sesamoiditis may arise. A dysfunctional hallux limitus may be the result of iatrogenic first metatarsal elevation (**Fig. 9**).

Many different osteotomies may be used when there is elevation of the first ray. Iatrogenic elevation of the first metatarsal after distal metaphyseal osteotomies may be managed by performing a plantarflexory opening wedge osteotomy (base dorsal, apex plantar) and inserting a corticocancellous bone graft.[19] Elevation is frequently associated with shortening. This combination is commonly seen after procedures performed in the proximal region of the first metatarsal (basal wedge osteotomy, lapidus arthrodesis). In that case, provided there is preservation of the first MP joint motion, a plantarflexory dorsal opening wedge osteotomy of the first metatarsal with preservation of a plantar hinge and bone grafting may be combined with shortening osteotomies of the lesser rays to restore the appropriate metatarsal parabola.

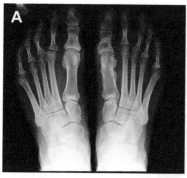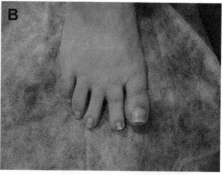

Fig. 8. Transfer metatarsalgia after hallux valgus surgery. (*A*) Dorsoplantar radiograph view shows shortening of the right first metatarsal. The left foot has developed Freiberg disease at the second metatarsal; compression of the second metatarsal head during the third rocker shortened the bone up to the point of reproducing an ideal metatarsal parabola. At the right foot, there is a second space syndrome with divergent second and third toes caused by an excessively long second metatarsal with respect to the iatrogenically shortened first metatarsal. (*B*) Clinical appearance of second space syndrome after first metatarsal shortening.

When there is marked distortion of the entire WB region of the forefoot (multiplanar deformities), pan metatarsal head resection of the lesser metatarsals and first MP joint arthrodesis may be the most efficient way to salvage forefoot function.[33] Once the first MP joint is fused, a straight line should be drawn from the hallucal interphalangeal joint to the fifth metatarsal, passing through the lesser metatarsals tips (3–5). This metatarsal formula allows for adequate forefoot supination in the transition to the third rocker.

Plantarflexion An excessive iatrogenic first metatarsal plantarflexion is rare.[19] In the presence of an excessively plantarflexed first metatarsal, midfoot supination with second rocker overload at the fifth metatarsal may be expected. Second rocker overload under the first metatarsal head combined with compression sesamoiditis will possibly be symptomatic. First MP joint dorsiflexion with or without plantarflexion of the hallucal interphalangeal joint will compromise conventional shoes. In this scenario, dorsiflexory osteotomy of the first metatarsal should be considered.

Others Keller bunionectomy was frequently associated with metatarsal shortening, first ray dysfunction, transfer metatarsalgia, and stress fractures of lesser metatarsals.[34,35] Revision surgery for a failed Keller bunionectomy usually includes first MP joint fusion and lesser metatarsal osteotomies or head resection. If there is no pain at the first MP joint and there is an index minus parabola, quantified triple Weil osteotomies of the lesser rays may be enough.

Lesser metatarsals
If focusing on the possible surgical procedures for the lesser metatarsals, several techniques may be considered for the management of transfer metatarsalgia.

Metatarsal head resection An isolated metatarsal head resection is rarely indicated in the treatment of transfer metatarsalgia. It would cause a load transfer to the adjacent metatarsal. However, pan metatarsal head resections play an important role in the management of the rheumatoid patient with a failed hallux valgus surgery.[36] If the failed hallux shows signs of arthritis and there are severe fixed deformities involving

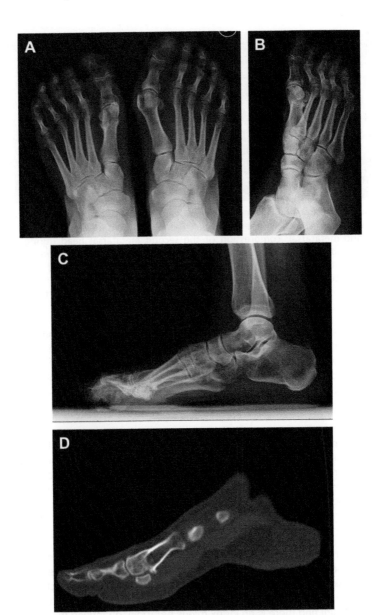

Fig. 9. Iatrogenic elevation of the first metatarsal head following mininvasive hallux valgus surgery. (*A*) Dorsoplantar WB radiograph view. (*B*) Oblique view. (*C*) Lateral WB view shows elevation of first metatarsal head. (*D*) CT scan confirms iatrogenic elevation.

all MP joints, the combination of a first MP joint fusion and pan metatarsal head resection could restore a pain-free forefoot (**Fig. 10**).

Condylectomy Although widely described, condylectomy has the potential risk of destabilizing the plantar plate that may lead to iatrogenic instability and arthritis of the MP joint.[37] Condylectomy may be used for the treatment of an intractable plantar keratosis, but condylar resection may lead to the transfer of the keratosis to the

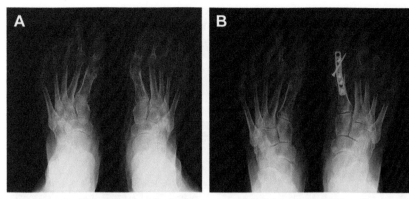

Fig. 10. Patient with painful forefoot after surgery. (*A*) Dorsoplantar WB radiographs with severe deformities involving all MP joints. (*B*) Revision surgery with first MP joint fusion and pan metatarsal head resection, 1-year follow-up.

adjacent metatarsal. A proximal osteotomy, a tilt-up osteotomy, or a triple distal osteotomy should instead be considered when looking for distal metatarsal elevation.

Tilt-up osteotomy A failed hallux valgus surgery may sometimes generate an axial metatarsal abnormal loading during the third rocker of gait. A transverse cephalic stress fracture over a relatively longer than ideal second metatarsal sometimes shortens the metatarsal to restore the ideal parabola.

However, acquired Freiberg disease sometimes generates a second rocker metatarsalgia and arthritic pain over the second MP joint. In those cases, a tilt-up osteotomy with a dorsal extra-articular wedge will restore the height of the second metatarsal head and allow for chondral reorientation (**Fig. 11**).

Proximal osteotomies Proximal lesser metatarsal osteotomy is a useful tool when elevation of a metatarsal is needed in the presence of a second rocker metatarsalgia. A dorsiflexion wedge osteotomy in the proximal metaphysis of an excessively plantar-flexed lesser metatarsal may relieve localized metatarsalgia. A proximal V osteotomy (ie, Goldfarb) provides fit of the fragments and affords good postoperative stability without the need of fixation. Immediate WB is encouraged to promote dorsiflexion and union (**Fig. 12**). Alternatively, a dorsal wedge linear osteotomy with screw fixation (ie, Barouk, Rippstein and Toullec [BRT]) may also allow for metatarsal dorsiflexion.[20] However, there is no way to quantify the exact amount of dorsiflexion together with each metatarsal individual motion in the sagittal plane. These osteotomies may lead to variable results and occasionally the transfer of a second rocker metatarsalgia at the adjacent metatarsal.

Cervico-cephalic distal Weil and triple Weil osteotomy Distal metatarsal osteotomies, such as the Weil and the triple Weil osteotomies, are designed to restore the ideal metatarsal parabola and redistribute WB forces around the forefoot. Repositioning of the metatarsal heads may be achieved through shortening, elevation, or a combination of both.

Weil described a simple technique to shorten lesser metatarsals in a controlled manner.[20] A single transverse plane osteotomy of the distal metatarsal allows a proximal glide of the metatarsal head. The amount of shortening achieved can be estimated by the length of the overriding distal end of the proximal fragment. The osteotomy is started about 2 mm distal to the dorsal tip of the metatarsal head and

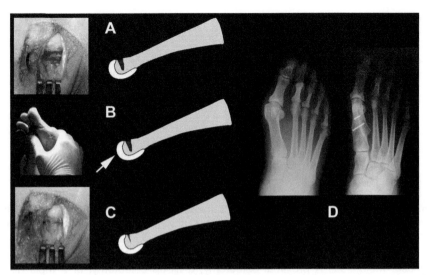

Fig. 11. Mild tilt-up/shortening cartilage-preserving osteotomy. (*A*) Dorsal extra-articular wedge. (*B*) Compression of metatarsal head to close the osteotomy gap. *Arrow* indicates direction of compression of metatarsal head to close the osteotomy gap. (*C*) Mild tilt-up and shortening of the metatarsal head. (*D*) Changes after scarf osteotomy of first metatarsal and tilt-up cartilage-preserving osteotomy of the second metatarsal. Note restoration of metatarsal parabola.

should run nearly parallel to the ground plane. With increasing declination angles, the head will descend, whereas with lower declination, the osteotomy cut will not exit the diaphysis. The correct inclination angle cannot be quantified; the surgeon must be familiar with the anatomy of the bone to follow the appropriate osteotomy plane. Originally, the osteotomy was fixed with a threaded K-wire. After surgery, the metatarsal should be unloaded during the third rocker. There is a risk that transfer metatarsalgia can appear in adjacent rays, particularly if they protrude distally with respect to the osteomized metatarsal.[38] The best way to ensure balanced loading of the whole forefoot during the third rocker is by reproducing the ideal metatarsal parabola, in which

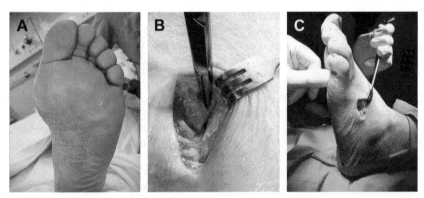

Fig. 12. Proximal elevation osteotomy is considered for the management of second rocker metatarsalgia. (*A*) Second rocker keratosis. (*B*) Chevron proximal osteotomy of the fourth metatarsal. (*C*) Metatarsal elevation.

metatarsal $1 = 2 > 3 > 4 > 5$ in geometric progression. When planning shortening osteotomies, the surgeon must assess how many metatarsals should be shortened and how much shortening should be achieved at each of them. Barouk[20] described the term "maximum shortening point" (MSP). It refers to the amount of shortening required at the worst deformed ray to unload it during the third rocker. A dorsoplantar WB radiograph is needed to design the surgical procedure. For example, in the presence of propulsive (third rocker) MP joint dislocations, the worst of them will mark the point at which the corresponding metatarsal should be shortened to provide for a relaxed reduction of the dislocation. Except for acute traumatic lesions, an attempt to bring the toe back to its original position (without metatarsal shortening) will likely fail in either the form of painful re-dislocation or a painful MP joint osteoarthritis. Once the MSP is established, the rest of the metatarsal heads should reproduce the new metatarsal parabola, so that it may be necessary to shorten more metatarsals. When determining the MSP, the fewer the osteotomies and the less metatarsal shortening the better, but sometimes all 5 metatarsals should be operated to achieve adequate correction. If there are no MP joint dislocations, the ideal metatarsal parabola should be reproduced with the MSP at the tip of the first metatarsal head. The MSP may be set at the first MP joint in the case of severe deformity after hallux valgus surgery. Adequate alignment of the first MP joint may require first metatarsal shortening up to the point where the proximal phalanx has retracted (**Fig. 13**). In the authors' experience, a 10-mm shortening of the first metatarsal is frequently needed and this amount of shortening does not apparently relate to the risk of generating a floating toe.

The results of Weil osteotomy have been well documented by several authors.[39–41] Stiffness is a major problem after Weil osteotomies.[42] Dorsiflexion at the MP joint is common in stiff joints, producing floating toes (**Fig. 14**). The following factors may be responsible for MP joint contracture[43]:

Existence of *extensor over-recruitment*. This phenomenon is linked to nonpropulsive metatarsalgia, in which metatarsal shortening is not indicated. Long extensor tendon transfer to the dorsum of the foot is required in this condition. Functional or anatomic equinus is frequently responsible for this compensatory mechanism.

Excessive metatarsal shortening that produces relative lengthening of the plantar aponeurosis may result in a loss of the reversed windlass mechanism, which provides the main plantarflexor moment at the MP joint.

Because shortening of the metatarsals is produced along the gliding plane, there is some amount of *coupled cephalic descent* with the original Weil technique. In the normal foot, the dorsal interosseous tendons (the only active elements that may provide for MP joint plantar flexion) cross the MP joint plantar to the joint center of rotation, which is located in the geometric center of the metatarsal head. After a certain amount of shortening, the center of rotation may be located plantar to the interosseous tendons, thus converting them into MP joint dorsiflexors.[44]

In the original Weil technique, the osteotomy is started at the articular surface itself to allow for adequate inclination. The new metatarsal head will have a *dorsal bony portion* and the total vertical diameter of the head will be increased. This combination may prevent the joint from providing full smooth dorsiflexion of the toe.

Since its first description, several modifications of the Weil osteotomy have been proposed.[45] By resecting a slice of bone instead of performing a single-plane osteotomy, the direction of the shortening will be coaxial to the metatarsal shaft and cephalic descent will not take place. The original relative path of the interossei with respect to the center of rotation will be preserved. Furthermore, the resection-osteotomy can be

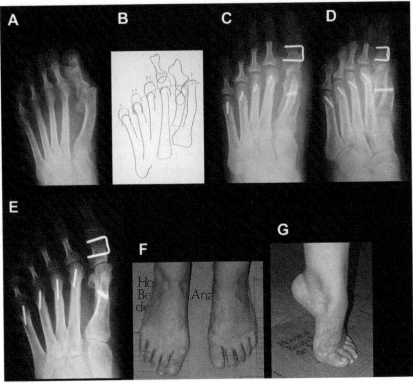

Fig. 13. Revision surgery after failed hallux valgus reconstruction. (*A*) Preoperative dorsoplantar WB radiograph. (*B*) Preoperative planning. (*C*) Postoperative dorsoplantar WB radiograph. (*D*). Postoperative oblique view. (*E*) Dorsoplantar WB radiograph, 5-year follow-up. (*F, G*) Clinical pictures, 5-year follow-up. Both motion and the windlass mechanisms had been preserved.

performed just proximal to the dorsal articular surface of the metatarsal, thus preserving the original shape and size of the metatarsal head. The resectional effect can be provided by both the double layer and the triple Weil osteotomies. The additional second cut in the triple Weil technique simply allows for easier control of the amount of

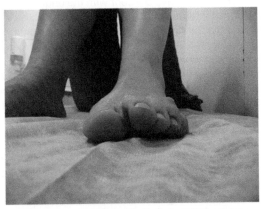

Fig. 14. Floating toe as a sign of a stiff MP joint after a Weil osteotomy.

shortening (**Fig. 15**). Risk of postoperative joint stiffness is reduced by performing resectional osteotomies.[43] Triple osteotomy decreases the primary stability at the osteotomy site with respect to the original Weil procedure because of the obliquity and the reduced contact area. This reason is important for the use of postoperative

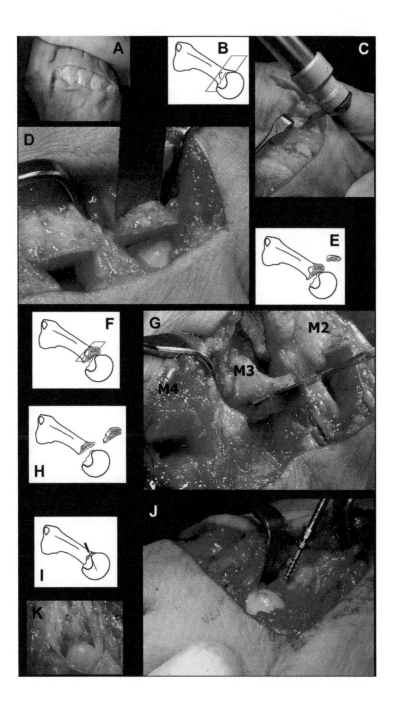

compressive plantarflexory bandaging for 4 to 6 weeks. The dressing will provide for rotational stability on the transverse plane and will help in preventing distal dorsal displacement of the metatarsal head.

Weil osteotomies may be fixed using 2-mm twist-off-type screws, 1.2-mm threaded K-wires, or 1.5-mm cannulated screws. Predrilling of the dorsal cortex of the metatarsal is advisable to minimize the risk of fracture.

Resectional osteotomies can be performed with minimally invasive techniques, where there is no exact control of the amount of shortening. Weil procedures without fixation had shown similar results to those with fixation when no quantification (assessment of the number of metatarsals and amount of shortening at each one) is made preoperatively.[46] Any cervico-cephalic osteotomy produces immediate shortening of the metatarsal. Many factors influence the amount of this shortening, including the extension of soft tissue release and the geometric parameters of the osteotomy itself. If no fixation is done, the ground reaction forces together with the immediate shortening factors will determine the final position and orientation of the metatarsal heads. Unfortunately, secondary displacement of the metatarsal heads is not uncommon after resectional Weil osteotomies without fixation.

Weil procedures are versatile, and medial-lateral shift of the metatarsal heads is possible (**Fig. 16**). If adduction of the toe is necessary, that effect can be achieved by displacing the metatarsal head laterally, and the other way around. Soft tissue release at the contracted side of the MP joint may be advisable as well, but there is no need for opposite side soft tissue tensioning; the postoperative tie dressing will provide for adequate alignment of the joint during bone healing.

Fig. 15. Triple Weil osteotomy. Surgical technique of the triple Weil resectional osteotomy. (*A*) The authors prefer the transverse approach just over the metatarso-phalangeal joints. After skin incision, blunt dissection is performed. Longitudinal arthrotomies are performed just medial to the long extensor. (*B*) Illustration depicting the osteotomy plane. (*C*) By plantarflexing the toes, the metatarsal heads can be exposed and the first osteotomy is made. In most of the cases, there is no need to release the collateral ligaments. The authors do not measure any inclination angle; the osteotomy is started just proximal to the cephalic cartilage and should exit the plantar cortex proximally enough to spare the insertion of the articular capsule. (*D*) The second osteotomy is performed on the coronal plane. (*E*) The second osteotomy sets the amount of shortening. This step is obviated in the double-layer Weil osteotomy. The mechanical effect of both double and triple Weil osteotomies is the same, shortening with elevation. The distal tip of the proximal fragment is removed. (*F*) The third osteotomy is initiated at the dorsal end of the second one. It is usually parallel to the first osteotomy cut, unless a rotational effect along the transverse axis is desired. (*G*) The authors perform the same step in each of the metatarsals included in the procedure; the picture shows a case in which all 3 osteotomies had already been performed in the second metatarsal (M2); the third one is being performed at the third metatarsal (M3), and just the first 2 steps are made at the fourth metatarsal (M4). Throughout the entire procedure, care should be taken to preserve the interosseous soft tissues. (*H*) The second bony fragment is removed. Its thickness represents the amount of elevation. This parameter is proportional to the amount of shortening and cannot be grossly modified. (*I*) After reduction of the osteotomy, together with additional desired effects such as mediolateral gliding, the osteotomy is fixated with the preferred implant. (*J*) Previous drilling of the dorsal cortex of the metatarsal is recommended for self-tapering screws. (*K*) Threaded K-wires are easy to insert. They should be cut at the level of the dorsal surface. In the rare necessity of removal, it is not much more difficult than screw removal.

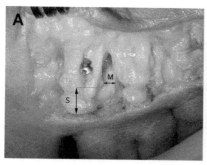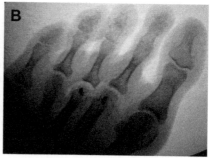

Fig. 16. Medial shifting of a triple Weil osteotomy. (*A*) Intraoperative view. Notice shortening (S) of the metatarsal and medial displacement (M) of the metatarsal head. (*B*). Intraoperative radiograph with displacement after screw fixation.

REFERENCES

1. Dockery GL. Evaluation and treatment of metatarsalgia and keratotic disorders. In: Myerson M, editor. Foot and ankle disorders. Philadelphia: Saunders; 2000. p. 359–77.
2. O'Kane C, Kilmartin TE. The surgical management of central metatarsalgia. Foot Ankle Int 2002;23:415–9.
3. David-West KS. Complications associated with Mitchell's osteotomy for hallux valgus correction: a retrospective hospital review. FAOJ 2011;4(3). http://dx.doi.org/10.3827/faoj.2011.0403.0001.
4. Kuo CH, Huang PJ, Cheng YM, et al. Modified Mitchell osteotomy for hallux valgus. Foot Ankle Int 1998;19(9):585–9.
5. Albrecht GH. The pathology and treatment of hallux valgus. Russ Vrach 1911;10:14.
6. Scioli MW. Complications of hallux valgus surgery and subsequent treatment options. Foot Ankle Clin 1997;2:719–39.
7. Lehman DE. Salvage of complications of hallux valgus surgery. Foot Ankle Clin 2003;8:15–35.
8. Espinosa N, Brodsky JW, Maceira E. Metatarsalgia. J Am Acad Orthop Surg 2010;18:474–85.
9. Espinosa N, Maceira E, Myerson MS. Current concept review: metatarsalgia. Foot Ankle Int 2008;8:871–9.
10. Kirtley C. Clinical gait analysis. Theory and practice. Oxford (United Kingdom): Churchill-Livingstone, Elsevier; 2006.
11. Perry J, Schoneberger B. Gait analysis: normal and pathological function. Thorofare (NJ): Slack Inc; 1992.
12. Maceira E. A systematic approach to the patient suffering from metatarsalgia. Revista del Pie y Tobillo 2003;17:14–29 [in Spanish].
13. Viladot A. Metatarsalgia due to biomechanical alterations of the forefoot. Orthop Clin North Am 1973;4:165–78.
14. Maestro M, Besse JL, Ragusa M, et al. Forefoot morphotype study and planning method for forefoot osteotomy. Foot Ankle Clin 2003;8:695–710.
15. Pedowitz W. Hallux valgus. In: Craig EV, editor. Clinical orthopaedics. 1st edition. Baltimore (MD): Lippincott Williams & Wilkins; 1999. p. 906–9.
16. David-West KS, Moir JS. Radiological assessment of tibial sesamoid position after scarf osteotomy for hallux valgus correction. Foot Ankle Surg 2002;8:209–12.

17. Chang AH, Abu-Faraj ZU, Harris GF, et al. Multistep measurement of plantar pressure alterations using metatarsal pads. Foot Ankle Int 1994;15:654–60.
18. Nigg B, Hintzen S, Forber R. Effect of an unstable shoe construction on lower extremity gait characteristics. Clin Biomech (Bristol, Avon) 2006;21:82–8.
19. Caminear DS, Addis-Thomas E, Brynizcka AW, et al. Revision hallux valgus surgery. In: Saxena A, editor. Special procedures in foot and ankle surgery. London: Springer-Verlag; 2013. p. 17–35.
20. Barouk LS. Forefoot reconstruction. 2nd edition. Berlin: Springer; 2005.
21. Silfverskiöld N. Reduction of the uncrossed two-joint muscles of the leg to one-joint muscles in spastic conditions. Acta Chir Scand 1924;56:315–30.
22. Hammel E, Abi Chala ML, Wagner T. Complications of first ray osteotomies: a consecutive series of 475 feet with first metatarsal scarf osteotomy and first phalanx osteotomy. Rev Chir Orthop Reparatrice Appar Mot 2007;93:710–9 [in French].
23. Jones KJ, Feiwell LA, Freedman EL, et al. The effects of chevron osteotomy with lateral capsular release on the blood supply to the first metatarsal head. J Bone Joint Surg Am 1995;77:197–204.
24. Garrido IM, Rubio ER, Bosch MN, et al. Scarf and Akin osteotomies for moderate and severe hallux valgus: clinical and radiographic results. Foot Ankle Surg 2008; 14:194–203.
25. Richardson EG. Complications after hallux valgus surgery. Instr Course Lect 1999;48:331–42.
26. Vora AM, Myerson MS. First metatarsal osteotomy nonunion and malunion. Foot Ankle Clin 2005;10:117–27.
27. Coetzee JC, Resig SG, Kuskowski M, et al. The Lapidus procedure as salvage after failed surgical treatment of hallux valgus: a prospective cohort study. J Bone Joint Surg Am 2003;85A(1):60–5.
28. Lapidus PW. Operative correction of the metatarsus varus primus in hallux valgus. Surg Gynecol Obstet 1934;58:183–91.
29. Trnka HJ, Zetti R, Hungerford M, et al. Acquired hallux varus and clinical tolerability. Foot Ankle Int 1997;18:593–7.
30. Tóth K, Huszanyik I, Boda K, et al. The influence of the length of the first metatarsal on transfer metatarsalgia after Wu's osteotomy. Foot Ankle Int 2008;29(4): 396–9.
31. Feibel JB, Tisdel CL, Donley BG. Lesser metatarsal osteotomies. A biomechanical approach to metatarsalgia. Foot Ankle Clin 2001;6:473–89.
32. Cicchinelli LD, Camasta CA, McGlamry ED. Iatrogenic metatarsus primus elevatus: etiology, evaluation, and surgical management. J Am Podiatr Med Assoc 1997;87:165–77.
33. Vandeputte G, Steenwerckx A, Mulier T, et al. Forefoot reconstruction in rheumatoid arthritis patients: Keller-Lelievre-Hoffman versus arthrodesis MTP1-Hoffmann. Foot Ankle Int 1999;20(7):438–43.
34. Friend G. Sequential metatarsal stress fractures after Keller arthroplasty with implant. J Foot Surg 1981;20:227–31.
35. Zechman JS. Stress fracture of the second metatarsal after Keller bunionectomy. J Foot Surg 1984;23:63–5.
36. Molloy AP, Myerson MS. Surgery of the lesser toes in rheumatoid arthritis: metatarsal head resection. Foot Ankle Clin 2007;12:417–33.
37. Roven MD. Intramedullary decompression with condylectomy for intractable plantar keratoma. Clin Podiatry 1985;2:491–6.
38. Bellacosa RA, Pollak RA. Complications of lesser metatarsal surgery. Clin Podiatr Med Surg 1991;8:383–97.

39. Beech I, Rees S, Tagoe M. A retrospective review of the Weil metatarsal osteotomy for lesser metatarsal deformities: an intermediate follow-up analysis. J Foot Ankle Surg 2005;44:358–64.
40. Hofstaetter SG, Hofstaetter JG, Petroutsas JA, et al. The Weil osteotomy: a seven-year follow-up. J Bone Joint Surg Br 2005;87:1507–11.
41. Vandeputte G, Dereymeaker G, Steenwerckx A, et al. The Weil osteotomy of the lesser metatarsals: a clinical and pedobarographic follow-up study. Foot Ankle Int 2000;21:370–4.
42. Migues A, Slullitel G, Bilbao F, et al. Floating-toe deformity as a complication of the Weil osteotomy. Foot Ankle Int 2004;25:609–13.
43. Maceira E, Fariñas F, Tena J, et al. Análisis de la rigidez metatarso-falángica en las osteotomías de Weil. Revista de Medicina y Cirugía del Pie 1998;12:35–40.
44. Trnka HJ, Nyska M, Parks BG, et al. Dorsiflexion contracture after the Weil osteotomy: results of cadaver study and three-dimensional analysis. Foot Ankle Int 2001;22:47–50.
45. Espinosa N, Myerson M, Fernandez de Retana P, et al. A new approach for the treatment of metatarsalgia: the triple Weil osteotomy. Tech Foot Ankle Surg 2007;6:254–63.
46. García-Fernández D, Larraínzar-Garijo R, Llanos-Alcázar LF. Estudio comparativo de la osteotomía de Weil abierta, ¿es necesaria siempre la fijación? Rev Esp Cir Ortop Traumatol 2006;50:292–7.

Treatment of Shortening Following Hallux Valgus Surgery

Andrew Goldberg, MD, FRCS(Tr&Orth)[a,b,*], Dishan Singh, FRCS(Orth)[a]

KEYWORDS

• Metatarsal • Osteotomy • Metatarsalgia • Brachymetatarsal • Arthrodesis

KEY POINTS

• Transfer metatarsalgia is a recognized complication following hallux valgus surgery in which there is iatrogenic shortening of the first metatarsal, especially in a Greek type of foot, which already has a relatively short first metatarsal.
• Management should begin with nonoperative measures such as shoe modification and orthotics. If these fail, then a step cut lengthening may be preferable to shortening osteotomies of the lesser metatarsals, which have risks of nonunion, stiffness of the lesser metatarsophalangeal joints, and floating toes.
• In cases of established arthritis of the first metatarsophalangeal joint, a bone block arthrodesis is recommended.

INTRODUCTION

Transfer metatarsalgia is a recognized complication following hallux valgus surgery,[1–10] usually as a result of shortening of the first metatarsal (MT), especially in a Greek type of foot, which already has a relatively short first MT.[1,2,10]

INCIDENCE OF SHORTENING AFTER FIRST MT OSTEOTOMY

The incidence of shortening following modern hallux valgus surgery is unknown, although certain surgical procedures such as the Mitchell osteotomy[11] or Wilson osteotomy,[12] by the very nature of their biomechanical effect, are more prone to give rise to symptomatic shortening (**Figs. 1 and 2**).

Conflict of Interest Declaration: A. Goldberg and D. Singh certify that they have no affiliations with or involvement in any organization or entity with any financial interest or nonfinancial interest in the subject matter or materials discussed in this article.
[a] Foot & Ankle Unit, Royal National Orthopaedic Hospital NHS Trust, Stanmore, HA7 4LP, UK;
[b] UCL Institute of Orthopaedics & Musculoskeletal Science, Royal National Orthopaedic Hospital, Stanmore, HA7 4LP, UK
* Corresponding author.
E-mail address: Andy.goldberg@rnoh.nhs.uk

Foot Ankle Clin N Am 19 (2014) 309–316
http://dx.doi.org/10.1016/j.fcl.2014.02.009
1083-7515/14/$ – see front matter © 2014 Elsevier Inc. All rights reserved.

foot.theclinics.com

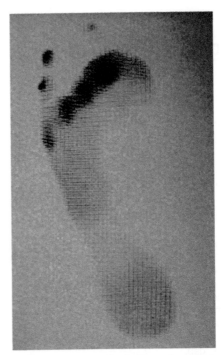

Fig. 1. Footprint of post-Wilson osteotomy for hallux valgus. Note the high pressure over the lesser MT heads, especially the second, compared with the absence of pressure under the first MT head.

WHEN IS FIRST MT SHORTENING SYMPTOMATIC?

Carr and Boyd stated that up to 4 mm shortening of the first metatarsal was acceptable in correcting hallux valgus.[6] Schemitsch and Horne concluded that a relative ratio of first MT length compared with the second MT length of less than 0.825% may cause

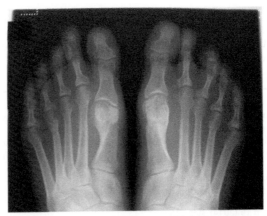

Fig. 2. A radiograph of the feet showing a shortened left first MT due to previous Wilson osteotomy for correction of hallux valgus.

symptomatic metatarsalgia,[2] a ratio that is in the lower normal range in accordance with Tanaka and colleagues.[13]

It is important to understand, however, that measurement of length on a 2-dimensional radiograph can only be part of the assessment, as the deformity is 3-dimensional; for example, dorsal elevation is not uncommonly seen after a Mitchell osteotomy. An assessment of a lateral weight-bearing radiograph will give an indication of the degree of elevation of the first MT head in the sagittal plane.

In normal feet, during the push-off phase of gait, approximately 64% of the total ground force is shared mainly by the first and second MT heads and by the tip of the hallux in roughly equal proportions.[14] In hallux valgus, the first MT can be relatively defunctioned, and more load is taken by the lateral MT heads, which can be restored toward normal loads by first MT osteotomy.[15–17] This is because in hallux valgus the first MT head is not loading through the sesamoids, which should sit beneath it. One of the aims of first MT osteotomy is to relocate the head back onto the sesamoids so it can articulate anatomically and bear load once more. There have not been any studies looking at the alteration of pressure distribution for different foot shapes or the changes in pressure distribution following surgical correction of feet with a brachymetatarsal.

CLINICAL FEATURES

The load-bearing area of the second MT is about half that of the first MT, and because pressure is related to load divided by contact area, the second MT is subjected to far greater pressures than the first MT, even in normal circumstances. In iatrogenic transfer metatarsalgia, the patient often complains of a painful callosity from shear forces on the skin under the second MT head. Patients have difficulty walking barefoot, and are limited in the shoes they can wear. Stress fractures of the second MT have also been reported.[18]

TREATMENT OF FIRST MT SHORTENING

The traditional treatment of this condition is by shortening osteotomies of the lesser metatarsals such as a Weil[19] or Helal[3] osteotomy. Weil osteotomies can result in pain or stiffness in the lesser toes[20,21] as well as a so-called floating toe, where the toe lies in an extended position and does not touch the ground; this has been reported to occur in up to 36% of cases.[22] Helal osteotomies have a high incidence of nonunion (up to 40%) and of persistent pain.[23] Although surgery to the lesser toes does have its place (see article on shortening by Maceira E, and Monteagudo M, elsewhere in this issue), when there is obvious transfer metatarsalgia as a result of a brachymetatarsal, the authors prefer a lengthening step-cut osteotomy when possible, or in the cases of an arthritic first metatarsophalangeal joint (MTPJ), a bone block arthrodesis.

Lengthening Step-Cut Osteotomy

The preoperative assessment of patients includes thorough history and examination; standard anteroposterior and lateral weight-bearing radiographs as well as oblique views are obtained. The authors find that the required information for accurate preoperative planning can be obtained from this assessment. They have not found that pedobarographs add any additional useful information.

The operative approach depends on the prior incision, but the authors favor a medial approach whenever possible. In this procedure, an osteotomy along the line of the shaft of the metatarsal is created with vertical limbs perpendicular to the longitudinal cut (**Fig. 3**). This bisects the metatarsal and allows for lowering of the MT head

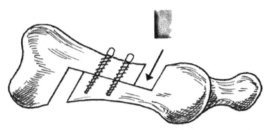

Fig. 3. Illustration of the step-cut osteotomy demonstrating a bisection of the metatarsal with straight and relatively thick bone segments. These are held with two screws ensuring the bone ends remain in a relatively lengthened position. Note the *arrow* indicates the location for the presized block of autograft or allograft.

and lengthening by osteotomizing in a plantar direction (see **Fig. 3**). In the authors' experience of using a Scarf-type osteotomy, in which the cut is parallel to the floor, the authors found that it did not allow as much versatility in enabling lowering of the MT head; additionally, the thin bone edges created were relatively weak.[24]

In the authors' technique, the 2 halves of the metatarsal are distracted by a pre-planned distance of at least 1 cm using a laminar spreader, and a presized block of autograft or allograft may be placed in the into the distal space between the bone ends (see **Fig. 3**). Care is taken to preserve the plantar blood vessels, which supply the neck and head of the first metatarsal. If following an inadequate correction in the initial surgery, lateral displacement is also necessary, then this is also possible in this technique. Once the planned position is achieved, with the bone-holding forceps in situ, range of motion of the first MTPJ is tested and compared with the contralateral foot. If necessary, a lengthening of the extensor hallucis longus tendon can be performed. If significant lengthening is obtained, the authors recommend that the tourniquet be temporarily released to ensure viability of the hallux. However, in the presence of normal vascular supply, the authors have not found this necessary for lengthening of less than 1 cm. Fixation is obtained by 2 compression screws from dorsal to plantar surfaces (**Fig. 4**). The graft may be held by compression in between the 2 bone surfaces, and a separate screw is only rarely necessary. Bone incorporation does occur without a bone block but is slower; the patient requires a more

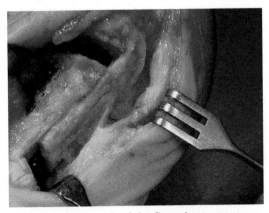

Fig. 4. Intraoperative clinical photograph of the fixated osteotomy.

prolonged period of protected weight bearing. If range-of-motion testing reveals the joint to still be stiff, then shortening of the proximal phalanx can also be performed. The increase in range of movement is achieved solely by planar shortening rather than a wedge excision osteotomy (eg, Moberg).

Postoperatively, heel weight bearing is allowed using a heel-wedged shoe, and providing tendon lengthening has not been performed, the patient is instructed on movement exercises of the first MTPJ at 2 weeks, with return to a normal shoe at between 6 and 8 weeks. Although lengthening of a normal first MT during initial first MT surgery may lead to stiffness, lengthening of an iatrogenically shortened first MT allows for a good range of movement of the first metatarsophalangeal joint (**Fig. 5**). The authors have found this to be independent of the chronicity of the iatrogenic shortening.

Singh and Dudkiewicz[24] reported on 16 patients who underwent this procedure with a mean postoperative follow up of 21 months. Four patients had a Scarf-type cut, and 12 patients had a step cut. The extensor hallucis longus tendon was lengthened in 5 patients, and a shortening osteotomy of the proximal phalanx was performed in 2 cases. Union was achieved in all cases at an average of 8 weeks. Dorsal tilting of the MT head occurred in 1 patient in whom bone graft was not used. Of the first 4 patients who had undergone a typical scarf osteotomy, 2 patients still needed insoles, and 1 patient subsequently underwent a Weil shortening osteotomy of the lesser toes because of inadequate lengthening of the first MT. At this point, the technique was modified into the step cut. In the step-cut osteotomy patients in whom inadequate lengthening (<8 mm) was achieved, the patients (n = 6) still suffered from metatarsalgia requiring an insole. When adequate lengthening was achieved (n = 6), all patients had good pain relief and returned to work (**Figs. 6** and **7**).

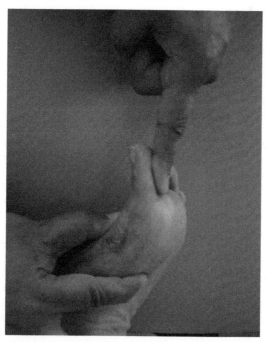

Fig. 5. Photograph showing the range of motion achieved after the lengthening osteotomy.

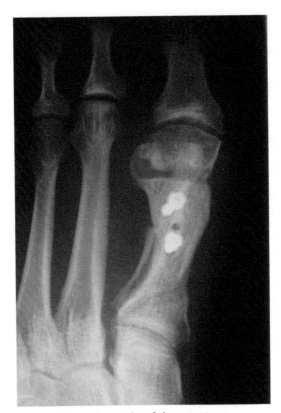

Fig. 6. Immediate postoperative radiographs of the osteotomy.

Distraction Bone Block Arthrodesis

This is usually reserved for patients who have developed arthritic changes in the first MTPJ. The incision is dependent on the incision used at prior operation. The joint surfaces are prepared for fusion by removal of any remaining articular cartilage and subchondral bone. Different techniques have been described that prepare the ends using circular reamers,[25] although the authors' preferred technique to create a stable configuration is to cut flat bone surfaces and place the bone block as a sandwich between them. The surfaces can be drilled or petallized with a small osteotome to ensure bleeding cancellous surfaces are obtained. A laminar spreader is inserted and the ends distracted until the desired length is obtained. The aim is to restore the joint surface to where they should be as planned preoperatively by assessing the radiographs, including those of the contralateral side. If there is any concern over the blood supply to the toe, the tourniquet is released and the laminar spreader left in situ for a few minutes while the bone graft is prepared. The toe should not blanch, and if it does, then a slightly shorter block might have to be accepted. A correctly sized block allograft, or autograft obtained from the iliac crest, is then placed between the 2 bone ends, which are distracted manually to allow it to be inserted. A firm flat surface is placed under the foot to allow simulated weight bearing to be tested and to ensure the tip of the toe clears the floor and can flex at the interphalangeal joint (IPJ) sufficiently to grip the floor. This optimal position is approximately 15° of dorsiflexion relative to the shaft of the first MT. Rotation is checked to ensure IPJ motion is in the

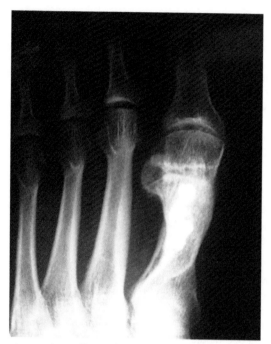

Fig. 7. One-year postoperative radiographs of the osteotomy.

correct plane and appropriate valgus is applied to allow the foot to fit comfortably in a shoe without rubbing against the medial aspect of the shoe or against the second toe. A 1.2 or 1.6 mm Kirschner wire is used for provisional fixation, and a 3.5 mm compression lag screw is placed from medial to lateral in the sagittal plane, followed by a contoured metatarsophalangeal neutralization locking plate, whose position is checked using an image intensifier prior to insertion of the locking screws. If the plate is used without the initial lag screw, plantar gapping can occur. Postoperatively, heel weight bearing is allowed (using a heel-wedged shoe), but no weight is allowed on the front of the foot until evidence of union, with the first check radiograph at 6 weeks.

SUMMARY

Transfer metatarsalgia is a recognized complication following hallux valgus surgery in which there is iatrogenic shortening of the first MT, especially in a Greek type of foot, which already has a relatively short first MT. Management should begin with nonoperative measures such as shoe modification and orthotics. When these fail, a step-cut lengthening may be preferable to shortening osteotomies of the lesser metatarsals, which have risks of nonunion, stiffness of the lesser metatarsophalangeal joints, and floating toes. In cases in which there is established arthritis of the first MTPJ, a bone block arthrodesis is recommended.

REFERENCES

1. Klareskov B, Dalsgaard S, Gebuhr P. Wilson shaft osteotomy for hallux valgus. Acta Orthop Scand 1988;59(3):307–9.
2. Schemitsch E, Horne G. Wilson's osteotomy for the treatment of hallux valgus. Clin Orthop Relat Res 1989;(240):221–5.

3. Helal B. Metatarsal osteotomy for metatarsalgia. J Bone Joint Surg Br 1975;57(2): 187–92.
4. Keogh P, Jaishanker JS, O'Connell RJ, et al. The modified Wilson osteotomy for hallux valgus. Clin Orthop Relat Res 1990;(255):263–7.
5. Pouliart N, Haentjens P, Opdecam P. Clinical and radiographic evaluation of Wilson osteotomy for hallux valgus. Foot Ankle Int 1996;17(7):388–94.
6. Carr CR, Boyd BM. Correctional osteotomy for metatarsus primus varus and hallux valgus. J Bone Joint Surg Am 1968;50(7):1353–67.
7. Stokes IA, Hutton WC, Stott JR, et al. Forces under the hallux valgus foot before and after surgery. Clin Orthop Relat Res 1979;(142):64–72.
8. Tóth K, Huszanyik I, Kellermann P, et al. The effect of first ray shortening in the development of metatarsalgia in the second through fourth rays after metatarsal osteotomy. Foot Ankle Int 2007;28(1):61–3.
9. Merkel KD, Katoh Y, Johnson EW, et al. Mitchell osteotomy for hallux valgus: long-term follow-up and gait analysis. Foot Ankle 1983;3(4):189–96.
10. Helal B, Greiss M. Telescoping osteotomy for pressure metatarsalgia. J Bone Joint Surg Br 1984;66(2):213–7.
11. Mitchell CL, Fleming JL, Allen R, et al. Osteotomy–bunionectomy for hallux valgus. J Bone Joint Surg Am 1958;40(1):41–58 [discussion: 59–60].
12. Wilson JN. Oblique displacement osteotomy for hallux valgus. J Bone Joint Surg Br 1963;45:552–6.
13. Tanaka Y, Takakura Y, Kumai T, et al. Radiographic analysis of hallux valgus. A two-dimensional coordinate system. J Bone Joint Surg Am 1995;77(2):205–13.
14. Hayafune N, Hayafune Y, Jacob HA. Pressure and force distribution characteristics under the normal foot during the push-off phase in gait. Foot 1999;9(2): 88–92.
15. Hutton WC, Dhanendran M. A study of the distribution of load under the normal foot during walking. Int Orthop 1979;3(2):153–7.
16. Hutton WC, Dhanendran M. The mechanics of normal and hallux valgus feet—a quantitative study. Clin Orthop Relat Res 1981;(157):7–13.
17. Nyska M, Liberson A, McCabe C, et al. Plantar foot pressure distribution in patients with Hallux valgus treated by distal soft tissue procedure and proximal metatarsal osteotomy. Foot Ankle Surg 1998;4(1):35–41.
18. Zechman JS. Stress fracture of the second metatarsal after Keller bunionectomy. J Foot Surg 1984;23(1):63–5.
19. Barouk LS. Weil's metatarsal osteotomy in the treatment of metatarsalgia. Orthopade 1996;25(4):338–44 [in German].
20. Trnka HJ, Mühlbauer M, Zettl R, et al. Comparison of the results of the Weil and Helal osteotomies for the treatment of metatarsalgia secondary to dislocation of the lesser metatarsophalangeal joints. Foot Ankle Int 1999;20(2):72–9.
21. Trnka HJ, Gebhard C, Mühlbauer M, et al. The Weil osteotomy for treatment of dislocated lesser metatarsophalangeal joints: good outcome in 21 patients with 42 osteotomies. Acta Orthop Scand 2002;73(2):190–4.
22. Highlander P, VonHerbulis E, Gonzalez A, et al. Complications of the Weil osteotomy. Foot Ankle Spec 2011;4(3):165–70.
23. Winson IG, Rawlinson J, Broughton NS. Treatment of metatarsalgia by sliding distal metatarsal osteotomy. Foot Ankle 1988;9(1):2–6.
24. Singh D, Dudkiewicz I. Lengthening of the shortened first metatarsal after Wilson's osteotomy for hallux valgus. J Bone Joint Surg Br 2009;91(12):1583–6.
25. Petroutsas J, Easley M, Trnka HJ. Modified bone block distraction arthrodesis of the hallux metatarsophalangeal joint. Foot Ankle Int 2006;27(4):299–302.

Index

Note: Page numbers of article titles are in **boldface** type.

Foot Ankle Clin N Am 19 (2014) 317–341
http://dx.doi.org/10.1016/S1083-7515(14)00039-4
1083-7515/14/$ – see front matter © 2014 Elsevier Inc. All rights reserved.

foot.theclinics.com

Moving?

Make sure your subscription moves with you!

To notify us of your new address, find your **Clinics Account Number** (located on your mailing label above your name), and contact customer service at:

Email: journalscustomerservice-usa@elsevier.com

800-654-2452 (subscribers in the U.S. & Canada)
314-447-8871 (subscribers outside of the U.S. & Canada)

Fax number: 314-447-8029

**Elsevier Health Sciences Division
Subscription Customer Service
3251 Riverport Lane
Maryland Heights, MO 63043**

*To ensure uninterrupted delivery of your subscription, please notify us at least 4 weeks in advance of move.

ELSEVIER

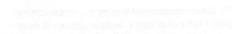

Printed and bound by CPI Group (UK) Ltd, Croydon, CR0 4YY

03/10/2024

01040487-0016